Introduction:
Time's running...

Sometimes I feel like a bazaar performer. I attempt to get everything under one rooftop and to satisfy everybody. There is frequently a ton to accomplish at work, particularly when the telephone doesn't quit ringing. At home there is the family including heaps of clothing brimming with shirts, which my significant other Martin was glad to press! (Furthermore I need to say, I like to do it as well!) The bills must be paid, the waste taken out and living in a perfect condo is a lot more pleasant than in a messy one. What's more in the nights I need to invest energy with my companions occasionally - and a brief period for myself would be great as well. Gracious indeed, I actually need to cook!

Today I need to acquaint you with the universe of solid, speedy cooking for experts. Also best of all, all plans are low carb and you don't need to have a blameworthy outlook on a bite!

I love my work, I love my family, I am extremely content with my life. But there were times when everything got a little too much for me! Even though my husband sometimes calls me a workaholic (and he's not much better at it!), I want to live a very healthy life. I attempt to do sports decently well and I need to eat steadily. At the point when you have a distressing regular day to day existence, in any case, it isn't that simple all the time. I purchased the espresso "to go" and the chocolate croissant unreasonably rapidly toward the beginning of the day - it goes so rapidly and tastes so heavenly. Then the same thing at lunch. I love servings of mixed greens and soups, yet sadly there is no flask in our office intricate and no solid eateries around the bend. That is the reason it's not unexpected a sandwich, pizza or other cheap food, contingent upon what your associates request! We don't want to cook for quite a long time after we get back home totally depleted from work. For the most part there is pasta, prepared dinners, snacks or whatever else is in the refrigerator. Assuming there was nothing at home by any means, we regularly requested from the conveyance administration, obviously you need to dive profound into your wallet in the long run!

Are you acquainted with that?

Don't stress, I was a year prior where you are currently and I can tell you: there is an exit plan! It is feasible to have a bustling existence and still eat soundly and not break your wallet! Martin and I got it done! In this aide, I'll show you how it works.

I'll show you how cooking turns into your companion rather than your adversary. The secret lies in the quick cooking! I don't mean fast food, but recipes that you can prepare quickly, but healthily and with few carbohydrates! MealPrep in particular (pre-cooking food for work) will make your everyday life and your conscience easier. Or more all, you have additional time since you never again need to stress your head over the thing you will eat each lunchtime.

I'll show you fast plans that you will love:

Everything is there, from bites and fundamental courses to side dishes. From exquisite to sweet treats and cakes, these blameless plans will spoil your taste buds. Bites and breads are likewise on the formula list! Also as a little something extra in addition, you get 30 plans for in a hurry: With MealPrep you can make a wonderful and peaceful regular life!

no time = stress

And additional time implies less pressure. How long do we go through each day worrying with regards to our food? An excessive number of carbs, such a large number of calories, excessively unfortunate? The amount of "food considerations" is presumably extremely high! Assuming you read "cook" presently, you will presumably ponder internally that you lack the capacity to deal with it. But I can reassure you: none of the recipes take longer than 20 minutes. 20 minutes, which you can take in the first part of the day and in the evening to get ready two or then again, if all else fails, even three suppers. But you can also take one day a week to pre-cook a whopping seven meals (MealPrep is the secret here!). Save yourself the psychological pressure and utilize the time saved to plan delightful recipes!

Let's get started!

But before I plunge into the flavorful universe of rarities, I need to reach out. I might want to disclose to you why you should utilize low carb in your regular daily existence and how low carb functions in any case. With low carb, various food sources are not permitted at various times or ought

to be
decreased. Why, why, why, I'll let you know immediately! I might likewise want to disclose to you what, notwithstanding time investment funds and a sound eating routine, the benefits of fast cooking are for you. I will likewise impart my tips and deceives to you, which will uphold you in your entire project.

Low Carb: What Is It About?

Low-carb is utilized as a term for some weight control plans: Atkins diet, New York diet, keto diet, ... Regardless of whether you are consuming less calories or for the most part following a low-carb way of life, the standard is something very similar: you eat not so much Carbohydrates but rather more fats and proteins.

What are high sugar foods?

Carbohydrates incorporate food sources like pasta, potatoes, bread, and rice. But don't worry, that doesn't mean you have to keep these foods off your diet forever. You should just ensure that you eat little of it or that you consume its better form: Whole grain rice, entire wheat pasta and yams contain more supplements and more protein.

Why truly do individuals eat little carbohydrates?

The principle reason many individuals keep away from sugars in their eating regimen is on the grounds that they need to get more fit. The less starches you consume, the fatter you can consume. What's more how can it all work?

This is the means by which low carb works

If you stay away from starches for quite a while, your digestion changes into a "starvation digestion". Whenever your body is at this stage, it is assaulting your fat stores. The way that your body has changed its digestion can make up for the absence of carbohydrates.

Low carb benefits

Not just the colossal weight reduction is a justification for why many individuals are as of now on a low-carb diet. There are various different benefits that I most certainly don't have any desire to keep from you.

Your heart says thank you!

Did you realize that sugars raise your pulse? Commonly, this proposes unreasonable fat utilization, yet sugars likewise assume a huge part and can prompt hypertension. Straightforward starches like white flour and sugar specifically lead to hypertension. It is smarter to utilize unsaturated fats and stay away from starches: LDL cholesterol is awful for your body, as it can prompt stopped up courses and, in the most pessimistic scenario, coronary illness. HDL, then again, is the "upside" cholesterol! So it's critical to consume more HDL cholesterol - this can assist with forestalling coronary illness. HDL cholesterol is found in unsaturated fatty acids such as linseed oil, walnut oil, hemp oil and also chia oil.

Protection against diabetes with less carbohydrates!

Sugar is poison for diabetics - that is no confidential. But this does not only mean that diabetics should only do without the granulated sugar. It is essential to by and large avoid straightforward carbs, as these comprise of sugar molecules.

... regardless of whether you are not a diabetic:

The more you consume sugar, the more your glucose level ascents. Your body then has to produce a lot of insulin in order to clear it from the blood. It is conceivable that sooner or later your body will arrive at its cutoff and can never again create insulin. That then ends in diabetes. So assuming that you eat less starches, you can keep your glucose level more stable.

The golden rules of low carb

1. Fat is your companion and not your enemy!

Carbohydrates are not terrible in themselves and critical for our creature. But if we then do sport and consume little carbohydrates, our body will suffer from the loss of energy at a certain point. This is the place where fat becomes possibly the most important factor: fat doesn't make you fat, it makes you thin. The main significant thing is that you pick the right fat. Look out for olive oil, eat a great deal of fish and don't stop at nuts and avocados all things considered! Sound fat gives your body significant energy and is a decent flavor transporter. What's more, fat assists with retaining your nutrients and supports your body in further processes!

2. Endless protein!

The less sugars you consume; the more proteins you need to join into your eating routine. Protein is likewise a genuine supernatural occurrence weapon with regards to getting in shape. The protein makes our body full or animates our organic entity to deliver satiety chemicals. So in the event that you eat a high protein diet, you will feel full for longer and can forestall food yearnings. Ensure your lunch is brimming with protein - this will keep you full for quite a while and avoid the evening low! Furthermore, enough protein guarantees that you separate muscles in your body more slowly.

3. Don't stop drinking!

Drinking is the most important thing in the world. What's more there's no need to focus on any beverages, however about water. The more you drink, the more you help your digestion and can consume pointless calories! Water additionally assists with purifying your body! We people are frequently dependent on sugar or gluten - that fulfills us to snatch a croissant and Danish baked good. The more water you drink, the better you detoxify your body and dispose of your habit in the long term.

4. Pay regard for your body signals!

I suggest that you eat three suppers every day, or possibly eat when you are eager. This will give your body sufficient opportunity to process. Our body is exceptionally canny and consequently lets us know when we are ravenous. Focus on this and feed him supplements when you feel hungry. Nonetheless, in the event that you've quite recently begun low-carb, ensure you're not reveling your sugar and carbohydrate

hunger. That is simply conditioning!

5. Colorful makes you lively!

Low-carb isn't just with regards to keeping starches low, it's additionally concerning what you eat, obviously. Ensure your food is pretty much as vivid as could really be expected. This doesn't mean sticky bears and know it alls, nonetheless a great deal of vegetables, including leafy foods. Search for a brilliant supper. In this manner you can guarantee that you have every one of the supplements in your body and don't experience the ill effects of withdrawal manifestations like exhaustion and food longings. With organic product, however, you should focus on the sugar content. You can partake in all berries, grapefruits, guava, citrus foods grown from the ground with a reasonable heart! We will meticulously describe the situation in the following chapter.

Foods You Shouldn't Eat

1. Bread and Grain

As a definitive provider of starches, you ought to keep away from bread and oat items later on, no matter what the structure: bread, bagel, flatbread or wrap: even the entire grain rendition contains a ton of sugars. There is no ordinary bread that has under 40% starch content. Rice and oats are likewise oats - so you ought to stay away from the two food varieties. Without gluten items ought to likewise be disregarded - sans gluten doesn't really mean free of carbohydrates.

I love bread and it is extremely challenging to manage without it! I subsequently prefer to prepare or purchase a low-carb bread with not very many starches. I use hemp seeds, flax seeds, chia seeds, eggs and significantly something else for this. It is vital that the bread "sticks" well.

2. Pasta

Pasta isn't just a staple food in Italy. In any case, to eat low-carb, then, at that point, you ought to eat less of it. A part of pasta has 91 g of carbs! There

is also hardly any fiber in pasta! Noodles are more of the empty, i.e. bad, carbohydrates. In terms of body feeling, pasta will hardly fill you up and satisfy you. When you crave pasta, it's just your conditioned mind.

Alternatively, you can change to zucchini pasta, additionally called zoodles. Then again, you can utilize different vegetables and utilize a twisting peeler to evoke vegetable noodles.

3. Muesli

Regardless of whether it is "sound" or not, muesli is high in sugars and you ought to subsequently eliminate standard muesli from your menu first. The low-carb variant consists of many nuts and seeds! But not only that: Spices such as cocoa and cinnamon can also give your muesli a special touch.

4. Legumes

Beans and vegetables are known to be high in protein and high in fiber. Beans and vegetables are sound, there's no doubt regarding that. But depending on which variety you choose, you have to make sure that some of the beans and legumes are also quite high in carbohydrates. White beans have 35 grams of starches, peas 41 g, chickpeas: 44 g, kidney beans 60 g carbs and lentils have 41 g carbs. So pick shrewdly which beans and carbs you choose.

5. Sugar and honey

Clearly: Sugar is an outright off limits, which you ought to stay away from with your low carb plan. But not only sugar, honey, agave syrup and maple syrup are also rich in carbohydrates. You ought to accordingly totally keep away from these variations! So supplant your sugar with stevia, xylitol, or other regular low-carb foods.

6. Milk and sweet yogurt

Milk has numerous supplements for your body. Calcium and B nutrients are fundamental for a solid eating regimen, yet you should in any case be mindful so as not to polish off a lot of milk. It's OK in tea or espresso, yet it's smarter to utilize almond milk for breakfast

or other dairy food varieties. Almond milk has just a large portion of the sugars contrasted with milk. With yogurt you need to focus on the sort of yogurt: normal yogurt is alright, however improved organic product yogurt from the refrigerated rack shouldn't be on your menu!

7. Juice and alcohol

Fruit juices contain a ton of fructose and furthermore a great deal of starches. Albeit the juice contains a ton of supplements, it likewise contains a great deal of absorbable carbs. Vegetable juices are the better decision: Opt for green juices and smoothies - these are nutritious and low in carbohydrates.

Caution: Even assuming a juice has a similar supplement thickness as a natural product, your body won't be loaded with it as fast. The sensation of totality is bound to set in with the entire organic product. So you better reach for entire fruit!

You must be cautious with liquor. Dry wine contains not many sugars, high-proof spirits none by any means. In any case, you should drink liquor with alert, as it will likewise make you hungry and hunger for starches and undesirable fats!

8. Vegetables high in carbohydrates

When you consider vegetables, specifically, you consider sugars. Thought wrong! Starches are likewise found in vegetables. Some have more, some less. You ought to particularly be careful with the sugar bombs. Eat minimal sweet corn and potatoes and furthermore keep away from parsnips. All things considered, you ought to eat a ton of vegetables as they will assist with controlling your glucose levels and forestall food desires. You can eat sufficient broccoli, asparagus, mushrooms, zucchini, spinach, cauliflower, lettuce, cucumber and celery. In the event that you're perusing this part, you're presumably thinking about what else you can eat! Relax, it doesn't imply that you will not be permitted to eat nearly anything from now into the foreseeable future. The response is: enough! I can let you know that much. Anticipate the delicious plans that are sitting tight for you in this cookbook!

Who is the quick kitchen suitable for?

On a fundamental level for every individual who is in the state of mind for solid low-carb food! The unique thing about quick cooking is "quick". Not at all like cheap food, the plans from the quick kitchen comprise of healthy and quality food sources. The speedy kitchen offers you shifted and scrumptious dishes that generally give you the energy you really want. Regardless of whether for you, your accomplice or your kids. We should have a fair eating regimen and that we get every one of the fundamental supplements. Our body is much more reliant upon supplements, particularly in upsetting circumstances! The ideal decision of food, along with clever using time productively, will constantly give you a solid, adjusted and, most importantly, tasty meal!

Tips and tricks for quick cooking

Breakfast for champions

Your morning meal is the venturing stone for the afternoon. Ensure that you have a fair and solid breakfast. Take opportunity in the first part of the day to begin the day intentionally. It has been demonstrated that "breakfasters" are fitter and more enthusiastic over the course of the day. Whether or not your life is unpleasant or not, on the off chance that you eat you will acquire energy - and consequently time - for the significant things in life!

Save time shopping

You presumably don't want to race to the general store and purchasing everyday food items consistently. That transforms the fast kitchen into an arduous one. Prepare of time. You can do a significant buy on more than one occasion per week. So you generally have every one of your basic foods prepared and you don't need to burn through your valuable time in the supermarket!

What's in your pantry?

Take a glance at the plans and think regarding which of these fixings have a long time span of usability. Nuts, eggs and significantly more will last a decent while. One time per month, plan a mass buy that will fill your storage space. Assuming the going gets tough,

you generally have something at home that you can use to invoke something!

Off to the cooling compartment!

You can likewise hold up large numbers of the plans! It has no effect while cooking whether you cook 2, 4 or 8 servings. You might have to clip somewhat more, however it essentially takes a similar measure of time. So for certain plans, simply cook twofold or triple the sum and put the extras in the cooler! Defrosted in the broiler or microwave, it poses a flavor like the first day!

What assistants do you have in your kitchen?

Depending on how you are prepared in your kitchen, it can also be that your utensils thwart your plans! Do you have a slow burner? Are your knives fuzzy? All of these things ensure that your cooking experience isn't too fun and lasts much longer than it should. You ought to have the accompanying utensils in your cabinet: pressure cooker, microwave, gas or acceptance oven, food processor, sharp blades, covered skillet and a hand blender or elite execution mixer!

MealPrep & how it makes your life easier

MealPrep is no confidential and has been utilized for quite a long time, however at last the pattern has a name as well. Rather than going out on the town to shop and preparing yourself a supper without fail, you cook every one of your food for various dinners. You can cook for one day (for instance toward the end of the week) and partake in the nourishment for seven days. Or then again you cook yourself a supper and eat something similar (or a somewhat altered variation) again for lunch the following day.

With MealPrep you generally have sufficient good food in stock, even in the most upsetting minutes. You no longer "have to" order from the delivery service or consume unhealthy frozen food (from the industry)! MealPrep is the solution for your weakest moments! The good thing about MealPrep is that you can prepare your portion - so you don't get the idea to take a   look. At the point when we are ravenous, we additionally will generally stack more onto our plates than we ought to eat. You additionally have your carbs and supplements under

control. You can design everything very precisely!

Are you hungry?

Let's begin and go on a culinary excursion! I'm truly eager to impart my beloved plans to you. My better half Martin likes it sweet, he likes to eat the marzipan potatoes. My top choices are the speedy shrimp curry and the zoodles with pesto - I like it more good. With these dishes you never again need to feel regretful - you can constantly eat strongly - in happy times as well as in upsetting times!

Note

I join extraordinary significance to the assurance of our current circumstance and have hence purposely kept away from photographs and pictures to keep the quantity of pages in this book as low as could be expected. This fundamentally helps the cost of the book.

In request to customize this piece of the formula and give it its own personal touch, I have saved some space for your notes where the space has permitted. Add any remarks, thoughts, or upgrades to make this book your own.

Please additionally know that a portion of the plans contain fixings that don't at first adjust to the low carb guideline. Nonetheless, these are utilized in such little amounts that the starch content of the completed dish isn't affected definitely and is still totally inside the cutoff points. With a low carb diet, 50g - 130g starches can be consumed per day.

The healthy benefits have been arranged with incredible consideration, yet are not ensured and may fluctuate. Except if in any case expressed, they allude to 1 serving (for an aggregate of 4).

Abbreviations:

l = liter
ml = milliliters
Tablespoon = level
tablespoon TL = level
teaspoon
Pck. =
Package g
= grams
kcal =
kilocalorie E
= protein
K = sugars F =
fat

Snacks

Minibulettes with yoghurt dip

These minibulettes are a hit at each party, but on the other hand are incredible as a nibble between meals.

20 minutes

Ingredients:

- 500 g of minced meat
- 2 carrots
- 1 red pepper
- ½ cucumber
- 1 onion
- 2 eggs
- 300 g of Greek yogurt
- 175 g feta
- 8 tbsp slashed parsley
- 2 teaspoons of gyros spice
- 2 tablespoons of bread flour
- 9 tbsp oil
- salt and pepper

Preparation:

1. First you strip the onions and cut them into fine cubes.
2. Then you heat 1 tablespoon of oil in a container and steam the onion blocks until translucent.
3. Meanwhile, add 4 tablespoons of parsley.
4. Then you put the mince in a bowl and blend it in with the eggs, the breadcrumbs, 4 tablespoons of yogurt, the gyros zest and somewhat salt to shape a homogeneous mass.
5. Now you heat up some oil in the skillet again and fry the minibulettes well on all sides.
6. They are then cooked over medium hotness for another ten minutes.
7. Meanwhile, strip the carrots, clean the peppers and cucumber and cut everything into coarse strips.
8. The feta is blended in with the remainder of the yogurt

and the remainder of the parsley.

9. Now you can serve the minibulettes along with the vegetable sticks and the yogurt dip.

140 kcal/7g E/11g F/2g K

Omelette with fiery prawns

This omelet rushes to plan and carries a ton of flavor to your table.

20 minutes

Ingredients:

- 12 shrimp tails prepared to eat
- 3 spring onions
- 1 clove of garlic
- 2 red stew peppers
- 1 piece of ginger
- 6 eggs
- 3 tbsp weighty cream
- 10 g butter
- 2 tbsp sesame oil
- 4 tbsp corn oil
- 2 tbsp soy sauce
- 2 tbsp lime juice
- 5 tbsp hacked coriander
- salt and pepper

Preparation:

1. First you strip the garlic and ginger and cut both into slender slices.
2. Then you wash the chillies and the spring onions and cut them into fine rings.
3. The prawns are split lengthways and, if vital, liberated from their intestines.
4. Now you put the eggs, along with the cream, somewhat salt and pepper in a bowl and combine everything as one well.
5. Then you put the spread and 1 tablespoon of oil in a covered dish and hotness the egg combination in it.
6. The egg should set over medium heat.

7. Heat the corn oil and sesame oil in a subsequent dish and steam the stew, ginger and garlic until translucent.

8. The prawns, alongside the spring onions, are set in the container and sautéed briefly.

9. Everything is then deglazed with lime juice and soy sauce.

10. The completed omelet is collapsed up and embellished with the prawns

11. At the end everything is sprinkled with the coriander

365 kcal/25g E/26g F/5g K

Eggplant Cheese Snack

This formula truly accompanies a preference for the vegetables.

20 minutes

Ingredients:

- 2 eggplants
- 2 tomatoes
- 1 camembert
- 1 teaspoon new mint, chopped
- 10 tbsp olive oil
- salt and pepper

Preparation:

1. First you clean the eggplants and cut them lengthways into 7 cuts. The external cuts are cleaved up and singed in a skillet with oil for around 5 minutes.

2. Then they are prepared with salt and pepper and pureed. The leftover aubergine cuts are sautéed in the skillet with oil for around 6 minutes and prepared with salt and pepper.

3. Now you put the aubergine cuts close to one another and cover them with the aubergine puree.

4. Then cut the tomatoes and cheddar into cuts and appropriate them uniformly on the aubergine slices.

5. The cuts are presently collapsed up and fixed with little sticks. Each part is burned again momentarily in the dish and prepared with salt.

6. Finally, enrich every one of the segments of the slashed mint. 149 kcal/5g E/13g F/1g K

Fine fish snacks

These canapés are appropriate for parties, yet additionally as a heavenly and sound nibble in between.

20 minutes

Ingredients:

- 100 g smoked salmon
- 400 g cod fillet
- 150 ml of cream
- 1 tbsp potato starch
- nutmeg
- 2 teaspoons of chives, chopped
- 4 tbsp oil
- salt and pepper
- 1 cucumber
- 1 pack of nursery cress
- mayonnaise

Preparation:

1. First you cut the cod filet into 3D squares of a similar size and afterward finely puree it along with a teaspoon of salt.
2. Then you gather the cream and the potato starch and blend everything into a single unit well.
3. Then you dice the smoked salmon finely and add it to the puree alongside the chives, pepper and some nutmeg.
4. Now you heat some oil in a skillet, shape little pecan measured chomps out of the combination and fry them momentarily on all sides.
5. The canapes should then prepare for around 8 minutes in a preheated broiler (180 °).
6. Meanwhile, cut the cucumber into strips and blend the mayonnaise in with the cress.
7. Then you put the fish snack on the cucumber and enhancement with a little mayonnaise and cress.

302 kcal/19.7g E/21.1g F/6g K

Baked spicy nuts

These crunchy and sweet-smelling nuts are not just delectable at Christmas time.

20 minutes

Ingredients:

- 300 g nut blend of your decision (low in carbohydrates)
- 1 lime
- 1 egg white
- 1 teaspoon salt
- 2 teaspoons of curry powder
- 1 teaspoon paprika powder, respectable sweet
- 0.5 tsp bean stew flakes
- 0.5 tsp dark pepper

Preparation:

1. First you crush the lime and rub the strip finely. Then, at that point, you blend the lime zing with salt, grind everything in the mortar and put it in an enormous bowl.
2. The curry powder, paprika powder, stew pieces, egg white and lime juice are additionally blended in.
3. Then add the nuts and marinate them well with the flavor mixture.
4. The nuts are then spread on a baking sheet and prepared in a preheated stove (180 °) for around 12 minutes.
5. After around 6 minutes you can turn the nuts.
6. Then you put the nuts in a bowl and let them cool down well.

487 kcal/14g E/40g F/13g K

Pear smoothie

This veggie lover smoothie is a reviving beverage between dinners. For additionally dazzles with its extraordinary green color.

10 mins

Ingredients:

- 200g lettuce
- 1 pear
- 6 tbsp lime juice
- some Tabasco

Preparation:

1. First you divide the pear, eliminate the stones and cut them into enormous pieces.
2. Then the pieces are placed in the blender and pounded along with the lime juice.
3. Now you wash the lettuce and cut it into huge pieces.
4. Then you put the serving of mixed greens and 250 ml of water in the blender and puree everything again very finely.
5. Finally, the smoothie is prepared with Tabasco.

46 kcal/2g E/1g F/6g K

Salmon canapes

These salmon bites are the ideal bite when you have companions over.

20 minutes

Ingredients:

- 100 g almond flour
- 100 g protein powder (neutral)
- 4 eggs
- 250 g of salmon filet, smoked
- 60 g cream cheese
- 60 g horseradish
- ½ cucumber
- 2 tbsp cleaved dill
- 1 lemon in natural quality
- water
- salt and pepper

Preparation:

1. First you put the egg white powder in a huge bowl and blend it in with the almond flour.
2. Then you separate 2 eggs and beat the egg whites until stiff.

3. Then add the excess eggs to the flour combination and manipulate everything with a little water and a spot of salt to frame a smooth dough.

4. Then overlay in the egg white with a spoon.

5. Now put some oil in a covered skillet and heat 8 meager flapjacks in it on both sides.

6. When the hotcakes have cooled, remove the bends on the right and left sides.

7. The cream cheddar is blended in with the horseradish and afterward spread daintily on the pancakes.

8. Now you separate the salmon cuts from one another and disseminate them uniformly on the hotcakes before you shower them with a little lemon juice.

9. Then the cucumber is washed and cut into dainty strips.

10. It is likewise dispersed on the hotcakes and all segments are additionally sprinkled with a little dill.

11. Finally, fold every hotcake into a roll and cut every one of them into pieces around 2 cm wide.

378 kcal/54g E/16g F/4g K

Zucchini Chips

With the vegetable chips you generally have a tasty and solid tidbit prepared that you and your visitors will like.

20 minutes

Ingredients:

- 800 g zucchini
- Paprika powder, blistering as rose
- 4 tablespoons of olive oil
- salt

Preparation:

1. First you wash the zucchini, remove the finishes and cut them into slender slices.

2. Then you line a baking sheet with material paper and spot the cuts close to one another on it.

3. Now you set a few salt on the cuts and let everything represent a couple minutes.

4. Then touch off the removed water with a kitchen towel and brush every one of the cuts with somewhat olive oil.

5. Now add a little paprika powder and heat everything for around 8 minutes in the preheated broiler (200 ° C) until the cuts are brilliant brown.

123 kcal/3g E/10g F/4g K

Grainy cream cheese with bananas and strawberries

This invigorating bite tastes great chilled and is especially great on pleasant summer days.

10 mins

Ingredients:

- 800 g of grainy cream cheese
- 250 g strawberries
- 250 g of bananas
- 4 stalks of mint
- some Xucker
- 4 teaspoons of new lemon juice

Preparation:

1. First you put the cream cheddar in a bowl and taste it with the lemon juice and some xucker.
2. Then you wash the strawberries and cut them into bits of the equivalent size.
3. Now you strip the bananas and cut them into cuts of the equivalent size.
4. Then you finely hack the mint.
5. Finally, segment the cream cheddar into little dishes, embellish with the strawberries and bananas and top with the mint as a topping.

205 kcal/27g E/2g F/17g K

Tomato and mozzarella antipasti

If you feel somewhat ravenous, you are erring on the side of caution all the time with these antipasti.

15 minutes

Ingredients:

- 300 g cherry tomatoes
- 200 g mozzarella balls
- 200 g olives
- 5 tbsp olive oil
- basil
- Chili flakes
- salt and pepper

preparation

1. First you wash the tomatoes and score them across at the foundation of the stem.
2. Then you put them in a pot with previously bubbling water, bubble them momentarily and afterward strip off the skin.
3. Now channel the mozzarella and add it to the stripped tomatoes.
4. The olives are likewise added and everything is showered with a little oil and sprinkled with bean stew, salt and pepper.
5. Finally, wash the basil, finely slash it and pour it over the antipasti.

322 kcal/10g E/28g F/4g K

Tomato and goat salad

The smell of ready tomatoes goes extraordinarily well with the fiery fragrance of goat's cream cheddar. For actually makes this serving of mixed greens so delicious.

5 minutes

Ingredients:

- 8 tomatoes
- 200 g goat cream cheese
- 2 shallots
- 4 tablespoons of olive oil
- parsley

- salt and pepper

Preparation:

1. First you wash the tomatoes and cut them into slices.
2. Then you wash and pluck the parsley.
3. Now you strip the shallot and cut it into dainty cuts as well.
4. Then you set the onions and tomatoes on the plates and spread the goat's cream cheddar over them in little portions.
5. Finally, shower the oil over the segments and sprinkle everything with the parsley, salt and pepper.

248 kcal/10g E/20g F/7g K

Greek caprese with olives

This tidbit is invigorating and sound at the equivalent time.

5 minutes

Ingredients:

- 4 mozzarella balls
- 4 huge tomatoes
- 16 Greek olives
- 4 tbsp hacked basil
- 4 tablespoons of olive oil
- 4 tbsp balsamic vinegar (date and fig)
- salt and pepper

preparation

1. First you wash the tomatoes, cut them into cuts and set them on the plates.
2. Then channel the olives and add them to the tomato slices.
3. Now sprinkle the basil over it and season everything with salt and pepper.
4. Finally, shower the olive oil and balsamic vinegar over the portions.

480 kcal/22g E/37g F/7g K

Italian caprese with Parma ham

The Italian variant with Parma ham tastes delectable and rushes to make.

10 mins

Ingredients:

- 4 tomatoes
- 1 parcel of rocket
- 2 mozzarella balls
- 200 g of Parma ham
- 60 g parmesan cheese
- 8 stalks of basil
- 2 tbsp olive oil
- salt and pepper
- balsamic vinegar

preparation

1. First you wash the tomatoes, basil, and rocket. Then, at that point, you cut the tomatoes into cuts and part them on the plates.
2. Then you pluck the basil leaves, cut the rocket into pieces and disseminate both on the tomatoes.
3. Then you cut the mozzarella into cuts and pluck the ham into pieces. For cheddar and ham are currently likewise conveyed on the plates.
4. Finally, sprinkle everything with oil, pour salt and pepper over it and rub the parmesan on all portions.
5. Depending on your taste, you can likewise include the balsamic vinegar top.

413 kcal/30g E/30g F/5g K

Meat dishes

Fried eggs with bacon, rocket and avocados

Also for the little craving in between.

- 8 eggs
- 2 avocados
- 80 g of rocket
- 120 grams of bacon

15 minutes

Ingredients:
- 4 tablespoons of olive oil
- salt and pepper

Preparation:

1. First you divide the avocados, eliminate the mash from the skin and cut it into strips.
2. Then you wash the rocket and serve it with the avocados.
3. Now you heat a few oil in a container and fry the morning meal bacon in it until it is crispy.
4. Then you set the bacon on the edge of the dish and fry the eggs in the middle.
5. Finally, set the eggs and bacon on the plates and season everything again with salt and pepper.

550 kcal/21g E/50g F/2g K

Bell peppers with sauerkraut and chicken filling

In this formula, the peppers are not loaded up with mince. The combination of poultry and sauerkraut, along with the yogurt sauce, brings about a truly scrumptious blend of flavors.

20 minutes

Ingredients:

- 300 g chicken schnitzel
- 155 g sauerkraut
- 2 red peppers
- 4 tbsp parsley, chopped
- 8 tbsp regular yogurt
- 2 teaspoons of mustard
- 4 teaspoons of oil
- Paprika powder, respectable sweet
- salt and pepper

Preparation:

1. First you wash the meat and cut it into 3D shapes of the equivalent size.

2. Then you flush off the sauerkraut and let it channel in a colander.

3. Now you wash the peppers, eliminate the seeds, divide them lengthways and fry them momentarily on all sides in a container with a little oil.

4. The meat is then burned on all sides in the hot dish and prepared with the paprika powder, salt and pepper.

5. Meanwhile, blend the yogurt in with the mustard and season everything with somewhat salt and pepper.

6. Now you add the sauerkraut to the skillet and, mixing once in a while, heat it up with the meat for around 3 minutes.

7. The combination is then filled the pepper parts that are still warm.

8. Finally, spread the yogurt sauce on the pepper parts and sprinkle with the cleaved parsley.

190 kcal/23g E/8g F/6g K

Ribeye pan with cherry tomatoes and avocado

Steak alone is a genuine involvement with terms of taste, however in mix with the avocados and delicious tomatoes it just preferences better.

20 minutes

Ingredients:

- 350 g ribeye steak
- 600 g cherry tomatoes
- 2 onions
- 2 avocados, ripe
- 4 tbsp parsley, chopped
- 4 tbsp lime juice
- 4 tablespoons of olive oil
- salt and pepper

Preparation:

1. First you wash the tomatoes and cut them in half.

2. Then you strip the onions and cut them into blocks of the equivalent size.

3. Next, you center the avocados, eliminate the mash

from the skin and cut them into bits of a similar size. Contingent upon your taste, you can shower them with the lime juice.

4. Now you cut the steaks into pieces of similar size and burn them on the two sides in a hot pan.
5. Meanwhile, season them with somewhat salt and pepper and afterward set them aside.
6. Now you utilize the browning fat in the skillet to singe the onions and tomatoes in it as well.
7. The avocados are likewise momentarily seared.
8. Then you add the meat and season everything again with salt and pepper.
9. At the end everything is sprinkled with the

parsley. 430 kcal/27g E/34g F/4g K

Colorful chicken vegetables in a wok pan

The vegetables from the wok are not just especially solid, they likewise taste extra crunchy.

20 minutes

Ingredients:

- 300 g of carrots
- 200 g bean sprouts
- 150g shiitake mushrooms
- 1 bundle of spring onions
- 100 g ginger
- 1 clove of garlic
- 500 g chicken schnitzel
- 75 g of salted, simmered peanuts
- 7 tbsp soy sauce
- 4 tbsp oil
- salt and pepper

Preparation:

1. First, you wash the fledglings and let them drain.
2. Then you clean the carrots and spring onions and cut everything into little pieces.
3. The ginger and garlic are additionally stripped and finely

chopped.

4. Then you clean the mushrooms and eliminate their stems.
5. Now you wash the meat and cut it into portions of the equivalent size.
6. Then you put two tablespoons of oil in the hot wok and burn the meat in it.
7. Meanwhile, season it with salt and pepper and afterward set it aside.
8. Now the carrots, garlic, onions, ginger and mushrooms are singed well on all sides in 2 tablespoons of oil.
9. After around five minutes add the meat, the fledglings and the nuts and keep on fricasseeing everything.
10. Then you smother everything with the soy sauce and 3 tablespoons of water, bubble it momentarily and season it one final time with salt and pepper.

450 kcal/43g E/23g F/15g K

Marinated pork steaks with green beans

The marinade makes the pork steaks in this formula especially succulent and spicy.

20 minutes

Ingredients:

- 450 g green beans, frozen
- 4 pork steaks
  - 2 cloves of garlic
  - 3 tbsp stew sauce
  - 2 tbsp soy sauce
  - ½ lemon
  - 2 tbsp butter
  - 2 tbsp oil
  - Chili flakes
  - salt and pepper

Preparation:

1. First, you put the frozen beans in salted bubbling water and cook them for around seven to eight minutes.

2. Meanwhile, strip the garlic, hack it into fine blocks and blend it in with a large portion of a teaspoon of stew chips, the stew sauce and the soy sauce.

3. The steaks are washed and afterward daintily covered with the completed marinade.

4. Then they are singed on all sides in a container with hot oil.

5. Then coat it with the remainder of the marinade and fry it for another moment.

6. The beans are sautéed with the lemon zing in hot margarine for around 3 minutes and prepared with salt and pepper.

7. They are then presented with the marinated steaks and, contingent upon your taste, sprinkled with a little gravy.

330 kcal/30g E/16g F/12g K

Schnitzel with Camembert topping

The combination of meat and cheddar in this dish intrigues and persuades each gourmet.

20 minutes

Ingredients:

- 250g chicken schnitzel
- 150g camembert
- 1 pear
- 4 teaspoons cranberries (glass)
- 1 tbsp oil
- 1 teaspoon butter
- salt and pepper

Preparation:

1. First you wash the meat, cut it down the middle transversely and singe it on all sides in a skillet with hot oil for around 3 minutes. Then, at that point, you season the meat with salt and pepper and set it aside.

2. Now you cut the cheddar into slices.

3. The pear is likewise washed, hollowed and cut into slices.

4. Then you heat the spread in a skillet and steam the pear cuts in it for around 2 minutes.

5. The cuts are then positioned in a baking dish and both the schnitzel and cheddar are put on top.

6. Everything is prepared in the preheated broiler (180 °) for around 5 minutes and afterward decorated with the cranberries.

380 kcal/37g E/18g F/15g K

Turkey skewers on a bed of lettuce

The sticks are extraordinary for your next garden party, however can likewise be eaten with the family in a comfortable atmosphere.

20 minutes

Ingredients:

- 1 kg of turkey breast
- 250 g lettuce mix
- 2 tbsp kebab seasoning
- 2 tablespoons of grainy mustard
- 2 tbsp olive oil
- salt and pepper

Preparation:

1. First you wash the meat and cut it into solid shapes of the same

size, every 3 cm.

2. Then you put the meat 3D squares in a bowl, marinate them with the kebab preparing, the grainy mustard, a little oil, salt and pepper.

3. Depending on the taste, the meat can soak for a couple minutes.

4. Meanwhile, wash the serving of mixed greens combination and pat it dry.

5. Now the bits of meat are placed on the sticks and burned on all sides in a container with a little oil.

6. Finally, you orchestrate the sticks with the

serving of mixed greens. 335 kcal/61g

E/9.2g F/1.7g K

Chicken breast fillets in lettuce wraps

These wraps needn't bother with any flatbreads whatsoever.

20 minutes

Ingredients:

- 800 g chicken bosom fillet
- 12 lettuce leaves
- 4 tomatoes
- 1 red pepper
- 1 green pepper
- 2 tbsp olive oil
- 4 teaspoons of natural soy sauce
- salt and pepper

Preparation:

1. Wash the chicken bosom filet and cut it into bits of equivalent size. Marinate it with soy sauce, oil and somewhat salt and pepper
2. Depending on your taste, you should allow the meat to soak in it for a couple minutes.
3. Meanwhile, wash the lettuce leaves and cut 4 of them into 2 strips each.
4. The tomatoes and peppers are additionally washed and cut into blocks or strips.
5. Now you put a few oil in a container and burn the meat on all sides.
6. Finally, put the cut vegetables and the bits of meat on the excess 8 lettuce leaves and season everything again with salt and pepper.

276 kcal/48g E/7g F/4g K

Tender pork fillet with bacon coating

Tender pork filet and zesty breakfast bacon.

20 minutes

Ingredients:

- 1 kg of pork tenderloin
- 600g bacon
- 2 cloves of garlic
- 2 teaspoons of lemon zest
- 4 twigs of rosemary
- 6 branches of thyme
- 4 stalks of basil
- 2 branches of chervil
- 80 ml of olive oil
- salt and pepper

Preparation:

1. Wash and slash the spices and put them in a mortar with the oil, garlic, salt, pepper and lemon zing and make a paste.

2. Then you eliminate the silver skin and the fat from the pork tenderloin. The bacon is put around the filet so that everything is covered. Then, at that point, brush everything with the spice glue and burn the meat.

3. Now you put the meat with the dish in the preheated broiler (80 ° C) and let it cook for an additional 10 minutes. At last, the filet is cut into cuts and served.

667 kcal/82g E/35g F/1g K

Stuffed peppers with chicken and vegetables

Peppers don't continuously need to be loaded up with mince. They taste extremely scrumptious even with this lighter filling.

20 minutes

Ingredients:

- 4 peppers
- 300 g chicken bosom fillet
- 4 cuts of cheddar cheese
- 100 g zucchini
- 100 g mushrooms
- 2 shallots
- 2 tbsp olive oil

- salt and pepper

Preparation:

1. First, you wash the peppers, cut them down the middle and eliminate the pips.
2. Then you wash the zucchini as well and cut them into blocks of the equivalent size.
3. Then you clean the mushrooms and cut them into bits of the equivalent size.
4. The shallots are additionally stripped and cut into fine cubes.
5. Now you wash the meat and cut it into bits of equivalent size.
6. Then you heat a few oil in a skillet and burn the meat and shallots in it.
7. Then add the zucchini and mushrooms, season everything with salt and pepper and fry it well on all sides.
8. The completed combination is then filled the pepper parts and covered with the cheese.
9. Then the peppers are put close to one another in a baking dish and prepared in a preheated stove (175 ° C) for around 14 minutes.

308 kcal/27g E/18g F/7g K

Baked veal schnitzel

A delicate veal schnitzel is likewise a genuine delight with each fundamental meal.

20 minutes

Ingredients:

- 4 veal schnitzel
- 400 g tomatoes
- 400 g of Gouda
- 2 tbsp olive oil
- paprika powder
- nutmeg
- salt and pepper

Preparation:

1. First you wash the meat and pound it daintily with the meat tenderizer. Then, at that point, you put some paprika powder, salt and pepper on a level plate, blend everything admirably and divert all the schnitzel from the two sides in it.
2. Now you wash the tomatoes and cut them into cuts of the equivalent thickness.
3. Then you heat a few oil in a dish and fry the schnitzel in it on the two sides for 2 minutes.
4. When you've turned the meat, top it with the tomato cuts and cheese.
5. Then the schnitzel and skillet are set in the preheated stove (200 ° C) and broiled utilizing the barbecue work until they are cooked.

592 kcal/55g E/40g F/3g K

Rabbit fillets with pesto pasta

A tasty and speedy low carb meal.

20 minutes

Ingredients:

- 400 g low carb pasta
- 8 bunny fillets
- 200 g arugula
- 4 teaspoons of olive oil
- 2 cloves of garlic
- 2 red chillies
- salt and pepper

Preparation:

1. First you wash the arugula and let it drain.
2. Then you center the bean stew peppers, strip the garlic and cut both into little cubes.
3. Then the rocket, garlic, bean stew peppers and olive oil are filled the blender and blended until a homogeneous mass is formed.
4. The pesto is then prepared with salt and pepper.
5. Now cook the pasta as per the guidelines on the packet.
6. Meanwhile, you wash the hare filet, season it with salt and pepper and singe it on all sides in a container with a little oil.

7. Then blend the pasta in with the pesto and serve it with the hare fillets.

490 kcal/88g E/10g F/13g K

Fresh asparagus with boiled ham

This exemplary formula is likewise reasonable for an eating routine in view of the low carb principle.

20 minutes

Ingredients:

- 2 kg of asparagus
- 8 cuts of ham
- 1 lemon
- cress
- some Xucker
- 50 g butter
- 6 egg yolks
- 12 tbsp white wine
- Two tablespoons of lemon juice
- salt and pepper

Preparation:

1. First, you strip the asparagus lances and remove the woody ends.
2. Then you put them in a pan with water, a teaspoon of salt and xucker and carry them to a boil.
3. The asparagus should now stew along with a teaspoon of lemon juice over medium hotness for around 12 minutes.
4. Meanwhile, put the egg yolks and wine in a metal bowl and whip them over a water shower until creamy.
5. Then you take the bowl off the water shower and liquefy the spread in it, mixing continually, until a sauce with a rich consistency is formed.
6. Make sure that the egg combination doesn't curdle.
7. The sauce is then prepared with salt, pepper and a sprinkle of lemon.
8. Finally, organize the asparagus with the ham, serve it with the hollandaise sauce and a little cress.

235 kcal/20g E/15g F/5g K

Chicken curry

A fast curry is consistently possible.

20 minutes

Ingredients:

- 500 g chicken fillet
- 1 onion
- 1 clove of garlic
- 3 tomatoes
- 2 tbsp oil
- 2 tbsp curry powder
- 425 ml coconut milk
- 250 g child spinach
- salt and pepper

Preparation:

1. Peel the onions and garlic, finely slash them, wash the tomatoes and cut them into 3D squares with the meat.
2. Heat oil in a skillet and fry the meat with the garlic and onions in it.
3. Meanwhile, add the curry powder and steam it for around 2 minutes.
4. Then you add the tomatoes, douse everything with the coconut milk and let everything stew for around 10 minutes at medium temperature.
5. Meanwhile, wash the child spinach and mix it into the curry.
6. Finally, season everything with salt and

pepper. 370 kcal/32g E/24g F/7g K

Chicken roulade with pesto

Pesto doesn't constantly need to be presented with pasta. It gives the chicken a delightful and delicious flavor in this recipe.

20 minutes

Ingredients:

- 4 chicken schnitzel
- 150 g pesto
- 2 tablespoons of olive oil
- 125 ml of vegetable stock

Preparation:

1. First you wash the meat and coat one side with the pesto.
2. Then you roll it up and hold it set up with a wooden stick.
3. Now you heat a few olive oil in a container and fry the rolls well on all sides.
4. Then you erase everything with the vegetable stock and let the meat cook in it for another 10 minutes.
5. Finally, cut the meat into cuts and serve

it. 212 kcal/37g E/4g F/4g K

Chicken fillets on orange salad

The fruity oranges likewise work out positively for poultry and give the dish a new, lovely aroma.

20 minutes

Ingredients:

- 600 g chicken bosom fillet
- 2 oranges
- 1 romaine lettuce heart
- ½ red onion
- 1.5 teaspoons of turmeric
- 3 teaspoons of olive oil
- salt and pepper

Preparation:

1. First you strip the oranges and cut them into their fillets.
2. Then you wash the lettuce and cut it into reduced down pieces.
3. The onion is stripped and cut into fine rings.

4. Then you wash the meat, cut it into wide strips and season it with salt, pepper and turmeric.

5. Then the meat is burned on all sides in a container with hot oil.

6. Then put the serving of mixed greens with the oranges and the onion rings on the plate and wrap the chicken bosom filets on top.

190 kcal/35g E/4g F/3g K

Lamb salmon on salad

Lamb is additionally reasonable for low-carb food and sometimes carries an extremely exceptional taste to the table.

20 minutes

Ingredients:

- 4 sheep salmon
- 4 teaspoons of hacked thyme
- 4 teaspoons of slashed rosemary
- 1 clove of garlic
- 2 tbsp olive oil
- 500 g blended salad
- salt and pepper

Preparation:

1. First you wash the meat and season it with salt and pepper.

2. Then you heat some oil in a skillet, divide the garlic clove and spot it with the open side in the oil.

3. Now you singe the sheep salmon all over it.

4. Meanwhile, add the thyme and rosemary to the skillet and rub the meat with it.

5. Then you eliminate the meat and let it rest for a couple of moments, enveloped by a little aluminum foil.

6. Meanwhile, you wash the plate of mixed greens and convey it on the plates.

7. Finally, you wrap the sheep salmon on the

plate of mixed greens. 224 kcal/32g E/10g

F/1g K

Lamb steaks with Greek style salad

Lamb steaks likewise taste extraordinary in summer when you cook them on the grill.

20 minutes

Ingredients:

- 8 sheep steaks
- 400 g of sheep cheese
- 8 tomatoes
- 1 cucumber
- 2 romaine lettuce hearts
- 1 modest bunch of rocket
- 100 g olives
- 16 capers
- 2 cloves of garlic
- 1 red onion
- 4 tbsp white wine vinegar
- 2 tbsp lemon juice
- 1 teaspoon chervil or oregano
- 8 tbsp olive oil
- basil
- salt and pepper

Preparation:

1. First you wash the vegetables, cut everything into scaled down pieces and combine them as one in an enormous bowl.
2. The olives and tricks are additionally blended in.
3. Then you mix the oil, lemon juice, white wine vinegar and oregano into a vinaigrette and season with salt and pepper.
4. The vinaigrette is now poured over the salad and everything is mixed again.
5. Now pluck the basil leaves from the tail, cut the feta into blocks of a similar size and sprinkle both over the salad.
6. Then you put a few oil in a skillet and singe the sheep steaks on the two sides while preparing them with salt and pepper.

7. Finally, the steaks are served on the salad.

460 kcal/45g E/30g F/8g K

Chicken liver pan

Liver has an exceptionally unique taste that makes its mark when joined with onions and peppers.

20 minutes

Ingredients:

- 600 g of chicken liver
- 4 onions
- 2 red peppers
- 100 g butter
- 4 cloves of garlic
- 6 sage leaves
- 4 straight leaves
- 2 teaspoons of slashed parsley
- salt and pepper

Preparation:

1. First you strip the onions and cut them into cuts. Then, at that point, you wash the peppers, eliminate the seeds and cut them into fine strips. For garlic is additionally stripped and cut into slim slices.
2. Now you wash the liver and burn it in butter.
3. Then you add the chime pepper, the onion, the wise and the inlet leaves and let everything stew over a medium hotness for around 5 minutes.
4. Finally add the leftover spread, season everything with salt and pepper and trimming with parsley.

203 kcal/30g E/7g F/5g K

Brussels sprouts pan with parmesan and ham

If you like Brussels sprouts, you will adore this skillet, on the grounds that the smells of ham and parmesan underline the taste even more.

Ingredients:

- 600 g Brussels sprouts
- 400 g of ham
- juice of one lemon
- 2 tbsp olive oil
- 80 g butter
- lemon meat
- 80 g parmesan cheese
- salt and pepper

Preparation:

1. First you clean the Brussels fledglings and afterward let them cook for 5 minutes utilizing the steaming tray.
2. Meanwhile, cut the ham into blocks and fry it in a dish with a little margarine and olive oil.
3. Then you also add the Brussels sprouts and mix everything together well.
4. While everything is browning together, add the lemon juice and lemon meat and season everything with salt and pepper.
5. Finally, set the Brussels sprouts combination on the plates and sprinkle all segments with newly ground Parmesan.

507 kcal/35.4g E/35.6g F/7.4g K

Veal meatballs with mushrooms

The minced veal utilized gives these meatballs an exceptionally extraordinary flavor.

20 minutes

Ingredients:

- 500 g minced veal
- 350 g shellfish mushrooms
- 6 sun-dried tomatoes
- 4 shallots
- 3 cloves of garlic
- 50 ml of white wine
- 200 ml of meat broth

- 200 ml of cream
- 2 tbsp chives, chopped
- 2 tbsp breadcrumbs
- 1 egg
- 3 tablespoons of olive oil
- ½ teaspoon bean stew powder
- 1 teaspoon paprika powder, respectable sweet
- salt and pepper

Preparation:

1. First you strip the shallots and the garlic and cut both into fine cubes.
2. Then you heat a little oil in a container, add half of the shallots and garlic shapes and sauté them until translucent.
3. Now you put the minced meat in a bowl and blend it in with the seared 3D squares, breadcrumbs, egg, bean stew, paprika and salt and pepper until you get a uniform mixture.
4. Then you structure eight meatballs out of it.
5. Then you clean the clam mushrooms and cut them into bits of the equivalent size.
6. The dried tomatoes are likewise cut into little cubes.
7. Then you heat a few oil in a container and fry the meatballs in it on both sides.
8. Then fry the excess garlic and shallot solid shapes in it and add the clam mushrooms.
9. The mushrooms are prepared with salt and pepper and afterward quenched with the white wine.
10. Now you add the broth and the cream and let both stew briefly.
11. Then the meatballs and the tomato shapes are added again and cooked with them.
12. Everything now has to cook for around 5 minutes.
13. Finally, taste the sauce with salt and pepper and embellishment everything with the newly hacked chives.

480 kcal/32g E/32g F/13g K

Crispy chicken schnitzel with kohlrabi

Kohlrabi is a particularly famous vegetable on purpose. Its taste goes impeccably with practically any sort of meat.

20 minutes

Ingredients:

- 4 chicken bosom fillets
- 800 g kohlrabi
- 200 ml of cream
- 200 ml of vegetable broth
- 1 egg
- 8 tbsp ground almonds
- 1 lemon
- 2 tbsp slashed chives
- 4 tbsp oil
- nutmeg
- salt and pepper

Preparation:

1. First you strip the kohlrabi and cut it into sticks of the equivalent size.
2. These are then cooked in the liner for around 6 minutes.
3. Meanwhile, put the cream and the stock in a pan and let them stew for around 10 minutes until a rich sauce is formed.
4. Meanwhile, wash the meat and season it with salt and pepper.
5. Now you whisk the egg in a plate and divert the schnitzel in it from all sides.
6. Then you turn the schnitzel in a plate with the ground almonds.
7. Then you heat a few oil in a skillet and fry the schnitzel in it for around 4 minutes on both sides.
8. The sauce is prepared with lemon juice, nutmeg, salt and pepper.
9. Finally, you arrange the schnitzel, along with the kohlrabi, and shower everything with the sauce.
10. Depending on your taste, you can sprinkle the segments with chives and wrap a couple of bits

of lemon close to them.

670 kcal/44g E/51g F/8g K

Tender fillet of beef with mushrooms

As far as taste, new mushrooms are basically past contest with a delicate piece of hamburger fillet.

20 minutes

Ingredients:

- 4 meat filet steaks
- 800 g mushrooms
- 8 shallots
- 2 teaspoons of oil
- 400 g of cherry tomatoes
- a few thyme, dried
- salt and pepper

Preparation:

1. First you clean the mushrooms and cut them into slices.
2. Then you wash the shallots and cut them into fine rings.
3. Now you heat a few oil in a dish and singe the shallots on all sides for around 2 minutes.
4. Then fry the mushrooms and onions for around 4 minutes and season them with thyme, salt and pepper.
5. Finally, you orchestrate the meat, alongside the mushrooms, shallots and cherry tomatoes.

355 kcal/40g E/19g F/4g K

Pork fillet with an herb crust

The spices utilized carry an assortment of flavors to your plate that you are likely not regularly used to from a pork tenderloin.

20 minutes

Ingredients:

- 450 g pork tenderloin
- 4 tbsp flour
- 2 eggs
- 2 tbsp parsley, chopped

- 2 tbsp lovage, chopped
- 1 tbsp oregano
- 1 tbsp basil, chopped
- 3 tbsp explained butter
- salt and pepper

Preparation:
1. First you cut the filet into 12 cuts and pat them flat.
2. Then you season the meat with salt and pepper and turn it in flour.
3. Then whisk the eggs and spices together and turn the meat in them too.
4. Then you heat the explained spread in a container and fry the meat on the two sides for around 6 minutes.

270 kcal/23g E/17g F/4g K

Fish dishes

Prawn tails with low carb pasta

The famous pasta is presently additionally accessible in a low-carb rendition. Along with the prawn tails, it makes a tasty and sound primary course.

20 minutes

Ingredients:

- 500 g of prawns
- 500 g low carb pasta
- 100 g parmesan cheese
- 2 spring onions
- 200 g of cherry tomatoes
- 2 tbsp butter
- 2 tbsp olive oil
- 1 tbsp parsley
- salt and pepper

Preparation:
1. First you cook the pasta in a little salted water as per the directions on the packet.

2. Meanwhile, wash the tomatoes and cut them in half.
3. The spring onions are likewise cleaned and cut into dainty rings.
4. Now you heat a few olive oil in a skillet and fry the prawns momentarily on all sides.
5. Then add the tomatoes and onions and fry them as well.
6. Everything is then emptied and set aside.
7. Now you pour the pasta and keep the pasta water.
8. Then you add the margarine and a scoop of water to the container, focus on the parmesan and let everything get hot.
9. Then you add the pasta and throw it in the sauce.
10. Finally, add the prawns, tomatoes and onions, heat everything momentarily and season with salt and pepper one final time.

430 kcal/25g E/20g F/36g K

Cod with a crispy crust

The fish in this dish is especially firm since we use almonds and dried up coconut for the breading.

20 minutes

Ingredients:

- 4 cod fillets
- 600 grams of broccoli
- 100 g dried up coconut
- 100g parmesan cheese
- 100 g almonds, ground
- 4 cloves of garlic
- 2 egg yolks
- Lime juice from 2 limes
- 5 teaspoons of slashed thyme
- 4 tbsp coconut oil
- salt and pepper

Preparation:

1. First, you wash the cod filets and pat them dry.
2. Then blend the parched coconut and almonds in with the egg yolk in a bowl.

3. The garlic is stripped, crushed and furthermore added to the almond combination alongside somewhat salt and pepper.

4. Now you put some coconut oil in a container and burn the fish on both sides.

5. Then you put the filets close to one another in a baking dish, shower them with the lime squeeze and sprinkle them with the coconut and almond mixture.

6. Everything must now prepare in the preheated stove for around 12 minutes.

7. Meanwhile, wash the broccoli florets and cook them still somewhat firm in the steamer.

8. Finally, serve the heated cod with the broccoli florets. 648 kcal/49g E/45g F/9g K

Grilled swordfish with herb marinade

The swordfish is extra sweet-smelling in this dish since it is handled with a spice marinade.

15 minutes

Ingredients:
- 4 swordfish steaks
- 1 onion
- One pack every one of chervil and dill, chopped
- 1 tbsp thyme, chopped
- 2 tbsp lemon juice
- 4 tbsp oil

Preparation:

1. First you strip the onion and cut it into fine cubes.

2. Then you blend them in a bowl in with the chervil, the dill, the lemon juice and the oil.

3. Now the fish is covered with it and left to represent a couple of moments relying upon taste.

4. Then you put the fish steaks in a hot skillet and burn them on both sides.

5. Finally, sprinkle the singular segments with the cleaved thyme.

330 kcal/50g E/14g F/1g K

Salmon fillets with green asparagus

This dish tastes new and fiery, particularly in spring. The green asparagus is likewise worth a pursue authorities who are not especially partial to asparagus.

20 minutes

Ingredients:

- 4 salmon fillets
- 24 stalks of green asparagus
- 8 tbsp olive oil
- 1 natural lemon
- salt and pepper

Preparation:

1. First you wash the fish and singe it on the two sides in a container with olive oil.
2. Meanwhile, cut the lemons into little boats.
3. The asparagus lances are washed and the dry finishes are removed.
4. The asparagus is then added to the skillet and furthermore fried.
5. Everything is prepared with salt and pepper and turned again and again again.
6. Finally, serve the fish, alongside the lemon wedges and the asparagus.

359 kcal/22g E/29g F/1g K

Prawns with avocado

In this dish, the prawns assume the principle part as far as taste.

20 minutes

Ingredients:

- 400 g shrimp, cooked
- 2 avocados, ripe
- 200 g cherry tomatoes

- 2 shallots
- ½ lettuce
- 3 tbsp lemon juice
- 4 tbsp balsamic vinegar, white
- some Xucker
- 6 tbsp oil
- salt and pepper

Preparation:

1. First you wash the avocados and cut the skin a few times.
2. Then you eliminate the mash from the stone, cut it into cuts and marinate it in a bowl with a little lemon juice.
3. Now you wash the tomatoes and cut them in half.
4. The lettuce is additionally washed and cut into scaled down pieces.
5. The shallots are cleaned and finely diced.
6. Then you blend the vinegar in with the xucker and taste the combination with salt and pepper.
7. Then blend in 5 tablespoons of oil and blend everything with the shallots.
8. Then you heat 1 tablespoon of oil in the dish, fry the prawns on the two sides and season them with salt and pepper.
9. Finally, blend the avocados in with the lettuce, the prawns, the cherry tomatoes and the vinaigrette and season to taste with spices.

500 kcal/22g E/41g F/8g K

Redfish fillet in a spicy mustard casing

The mustard covering gives the fish filet not simply one

20 minutes

Ingredients:

- 750 g redfish fillet
- 2 eggs
- 100 g breadcrumbs
- 5 tbsp flour
- 150g salad

- 2 tbsp mustard
- 2 tbsp balsamic vinegar, white
- 1 teaspoon lemon juice
- 4 tbsp rapeseed oil
- salt and pepper

Preparation:

1. First you wash the lettuce and let it dry.
2. Then blend 1 tablespoon of mustard in with the vinegar and lemon juice and furthermore overlap in two tablespoons of oil.
3. Presently the vinaigrette is prepared with salt and pepper and blended in with the serving of mixed greens. Then, at that point, flush the fish, partition it into 4 pieces and season it with salt and pepper.
4. The eggs are then rushed with a tablespoon of mustard.
5. The filets are presently cleaned with flour, then, at that point, turned first in the egg-mustard blend and afterward in the breadcrumbs, and

then singed in 2 tablespoons of oil for around 4 minutes.

6. The fish is presented with the plate

of mixed greens. for kcal/38g

E/20g F/14g K

Salmon with crab meat filling

These nibbles are the ideal thing for fish lovers.

20 minutes

Ingredients:

- 8 cuts of smoked salmon
- 350g crab meat
- 12 lettuce leaves
- 150 ml of cream
- 4 teaspoons of horseradish
- 1 tbsp lemon juice
- 1 lemon
- 2 branches of dill

- salt and pepper

Preparation:

1. First you wash the lettuce leaves and convey them on the four plates.
2. Then whip the cream until solid, taste it with a little lemon squeeze and blend it in with the horseradish.
3. Now you add the crab meat, mix everything great and season it with salt and pepper.
4. The crab meat blend is currently circulated on the salmon cuts, everything is moved up and fixed with a wooden skewer.
5. The fish chomps are then spread over the lettuce leaves and embellished with a couple of lemon wedges and a little dill.

250 kcal/25g E/15g F/3g K

Shrimp pan on fire

This shrimp container will carry a ton of fire to your table.

20 minutes

Ingredients:

- 400g prawns, prepared to eat
- 300g cherry tomatoes
- 3 zucchini
- 5 cloves of garlic
- 1 bundle of spring onions
- 3 stew peppers
- 6 tbsp slashed parsley
- 3 tablespoons of olive oil
- salt and pepper

Preparation:

1. First you wash the zucchini and cut them into bits of the equivalent size.
2. Then you clean the spring onions and cut them into fine rings.
3. Then you strip the garlic and cut the cloves in 2 halves.
4. The bean stew peppers are likewise washed and cut into fine strips.

5. Then put 2 tablespoons of oil in a skillet and fry the prawns energetically on all sides.
6. They are then removed from the dish and set aside.
7. Now add one more tablespoon of oil to the dish and fry the spring onions and zucchini well on all sides.
8. Then you add the garlic, the stew peppers and the cherry tomatoes and keep on broiling everything together.
9. Then the prawns are added and everything is prepared again with salt and pepper.
10. Finally, sprinkle the shrimp skillet with the new parsley.

190 kcal/22g E/7g F/10g K

Salmon fillet on a bed of leeks

The sweet-smelling salmon and the zest of the leek bring about a delectable mix of flavors in this dish.

20 minutes

Ingredients:

- 4 salmon fillets
- 1 yellow pepper
- 2 leeks
- 1 onion
- 100 g harsh cream
- 2 tbsp oil
- Paprika powder, respectable sweet
- Xucker
- salt and pepper

Preparation:

1. First you wash the peppers and cut them into little cubes.
2. Then you wash the leek and cut it into fine rings.
3. The onion is additionally stripped and cut into blocks of the equivalent size.
4. Then you wash the fish and season it with salt and pepper.
5. Then you heat 1 tablespoon of oil in the container and singe the peppers and onions on all sides.
6. The leek is additionally added and burned briefly.

7. Now you add the cream, mix everything admirably and taste it with pepper and xucker.

8. Everything must now stew for around 4 minutes.

9. Meanwhile, heat 1 tablespoon of oil in one more skillet and fry the fish in it over medium hotness for around 5 minutes on all sides.

10. Then the vegetables are prepared with the paprika powder.

11. Finally, set the vegetables on the plate and put the salmon on top.

12. Depending on your taste, you can prepare again with a little paprika powder.

350 kcal/28g E/25g F/5g K

Salmon fillet with a refreshing cucumber ragout

In this formula, the salmon, in mix with the cucumber combination, has an especially invigorating aroma.

20 minutes

Ingredients:

- 500 g salmon fillet
- 1 kg of cucumber
- 1 onion
- 150 g cream cheddar with horseradish
- 1 teaspoon vegetable stock
- 2 tbsp sauce thickener, light
- 4 teaspoons of dill, chopped
- 3 tbsp oil
- salt and pepper

Preparation:

1. First you wash the salmon and cut it into 3D shapes of the equivalent size.

2. Then you heat 2 tablespoons of oil in a dish and singe the fish on all sides.

3. Now you strip the cucumbers and divide them lengthways so you can eliminate the seeds.

4. Then you cut them into even slices.

5. Then you strip the onion and cut it into fine cubes.

6. The completed salmon is prepared with salt and eliminated from the pan.

7. Then hotness up 1 tablespoon of oil again and fry the cucumbers and onions in it.

8. Then you stifle both with 250 ml of water, add the teaspoon vegetable stock and mix in the cream cheese.

9. Everything is briefly boiled and then simmered for around 7 minutes.

10. Then thicken everything with a little sauce thickener and season it again with salt and pepper.

11. Finally, the salmon is lifted into the cucumber blend and everything is decorated with the cleaved dill.

450 kcal/28g E/33g F/8g K

Quick curry with prawns and coconut

A colorful variation of the curry 20 minutes

Ingredients:

- 400 g of prawns, prepared to eat
- 200 g cherry tomatoes
- 1 bean stew pepper
- 1 jar of coconut milk, unsweetened
- 2 tbsp hacked coriander
- 1 lime
- 1 tbsp oil
- curry powder
- Xucker

Preparation:

1. First you wash the tomatoes and cut them in half.

2. Then you wash the stew, cut it into fine 3D squares and sauté it momentarily in a pan with 2 teaspoons of curry.

3. Then you add the coconut milk and 1/8 liter of water to the pot, bubble everything momentarily and season it with 1/2 teaspoon of salt and 1 teaspoon of Xucker.

4. Then you add the tomatoes and the prawns and let everything stew for around 5 minutes.

5. Meanwhile, crush the lime and taste the curry with the juice and a little salt.

6. Finally, add the hacked coriander to the individual servings.

280 kcal/20g E/19g F/6g K

Asian style salmon with spinach

The soy sauce utilized gives the salmon a marginally pungent and zesty taste and goes impeccably with asparagus.

20 minutes

Ingredients:

- 600 g of salmon
- 800 g of spinach
- 4 spring onions
- 4 teaspoons of oil
- 200 ml of vegetable broth
- 4 tsp soy sauce
- 4 teaspoons of ginger, diced
- salt and pepper

Preparation:

1. First you wash the onions and cut them into fine rings and fry them in a little oil in a pan.

2. Now you put the salmon filet in the dish, fry it on the two sides and afterward set it aside.

3. Now the spinach is warmed in the searing fat until it collapses.

4. Meanwhile, season it with salt and pepper and steadily add the vegetable stock, soy sauce and ginger.

5. Finally, set the salmon back in the container and let everything cook for an additional 3 minutes with the top closed.

365 kcal/39g E/20g F/4g K

Grilled cod with herbs and tomatoes

Cod is an exceptionally famous fish which is as it should be. Along with the spices and the fruity tomatoes, a reviving dish is created.

20 minutes

Ingredients:

- 4 cod fillets
- 800 g cherry tomatoes
- 4 tbsp butter
- 4 tbsp oil
- 4 tbsp slashed basil
- juice of one lemon
- salt and pepper

Preparation:

1. First, you wash the fish and pat it dry.
2. Then you wash the tomatoes and cut them in half.
3. Then you heat a few margarine and oil in a container and singe the cod filets on both sides.
4. Meanwhile, season them with salt and pepper.
5. Then the tomatoes and basil are added to the skillet until everything is hot.
6. Finally, pour the lemon juice over the fish and orchestrate everything together.

445 kcal/44g E/28g F/3g K

Salmon fillet with thyme

Thyme is perhaps the most tasty spice and goes impeccably with the smell of the fish.

20 minutes

Ingredients:

- 4 salmon fillets
- 1 pack of thyme
- 2 natural lemons
- 2 cloves of garlic
- 2 tbsp oil
- 2 tbsp butter

- salt and pepper

Preparation:

1. First you wash the fish, pluck the thyme and cleave it up. The garlic is stripped and halved.
2. Then you wash the lemon and cut it into slices.
3. Now you heat a few oil and margarine in a dish and spot the garlic parts with the cut side in the fat.
4. The salmon steaks are prepared with salt, pepper and thyme and afterward positioned in the pan.
5. Everything is burned for a few minutes before the salmon is turned.
6. After turning, cover the highest point of the fish with the lemon cuts, put the container in the preheated (160 ° C fan stove) for around 10 minutes and let it cook.

300 kcal/40g E/15g F/0g K

Low carb bread with trout and avocado cream

A decent option for a fundamental meal.

10 mins

Ingredients:

- 8 cuts of low carb bread
- 1 avocado
- 150g smoked trout
- 2 tbsp cress
- 40 g of strawberry jelly
- 1 lemon
- 1 red chilli
- salt and pepper

Preparation:

1. First you split the avocados, eliminate the mash from the skin and crush it into a velvety mass.
2. You currently spread this combination onto the bread slices.
3. The trout is likewise culled into little pieces with a fork and put on the avocado cream.
4. Now you can sprinkle the cress over the portions.

5. The lemon is pressed and the bean stew pepper is divided, hollowed and slashed into fine pieces.

6. Now blend the strawberry jam with a little lemon squeeze, the chillies and salt and pepper.

7. The strawberry combination is then added to the bread as a topping.

425 kcal/21g E/33g F/9g K

Tuna in herb crust

This formula is additionally really great for the barbecue. For spices utilized give the fish a fine flavor.

20 minutes

Ingredients:

- 4 fish steaks á 200 g
- 2 natural lemons
- 4 tbsp sesame oil
- 1 teaspoon rosemary, chopped
- 1 teaspoon thyme, chopped
- 2 bean stew peppers
- 2 cloves of garlic
- 4 tbsp sesame oil
- 2 tbsp pink berries
- 2 teaspoons of lemon zest
- salt

Preparation:

1. First, you wash the fish and pat it dry.

2. Then you wash the lemons, rub the strips, and cut the mash into slices.

3. Then split the stew peppers, center them and hack them up.

4. The garlic is additionally stripped and cut into fine cubes.

5. Now put the rosemary and thyme, along with the lemon zing, garlic, bean stew peppers, pink berries, salt and sesame oil in a bowl and pulverize everything well.

6. Then you heat the sesame oil in a skillet and burn the fish steaks on both sides.

7. Then you set the spice blend on the steaks and give them along with the lemon wedges for around 8 minutes in the preheated stove (120 ° C).

377 kcal/44g E/22g F/1g K

Vegetarian / vegan

Chilled vegetable soup

This soup is a genuine delight for vegetable fans.

20 minutes

Ingredients:

- 2 green peppers
- 2 carrots
- 2 cucumbers
- 4 spring onions
- 3 stems of celery
- 300 ml natural tomato juice
- 50 ml of olive oil
- Tabasco
- salt and pepper

Preparation:

1. First you eliminate the skin of the cucumber, cut it down the middle lengthways and eliminate the seeds with a spoon.
2. Wash the peppers, eliminate the seeds and cut them into little pieces with the stripped carrots.
3. Now cleave and wash the celery and spring onions
4. Now every one of the vegetables are placed in a blender and finely pureed.
5. The puree is then blended in with the tomato squeeze and oil and prepared with salt, pepper and Tabasco.

110 kcal/5g E/7g F/8g K

Quick cheese salad

With this formula you can invoke a genuine delight for genuine cheddar fans in 20 minutes.

15 minutes

Ingredients:

- 400 g of rancher's cheese
- 200 g pickles
- 4 tbsp slashed parsley
- 1 oak leaf salad
- 2 red onions
- 6 tbsp white wine vinegar
- 1 teaspoon mustard
- some Xucker
- 4 tbsp oil
- salt and pepper

Preparation:

1. First you put the vinegar in a bowl and blend it in with the mustard, the xucker, the oil and somewhat salt and pepper.
2. Then you strip the onions, cut them into little shapes and blend them in with the vinaigrette.
3. Now you wash the lettuce and cut it into nibble sized pieces.
4. The cucumbers are likewise cut into slim slices.
5. Then cut the cheddar into fine strips.
6. Finally, blend the lettuce, cucumber and cheddar with the vinaigrette and trimming everything with the parsley.

520 kcal/29g E/40g F/7g K

Roman style mozzarella salad

This salad is speedy and simple to get ready and tastes extraordinary as a primary supper or snack.

15 minutes

Ingredients:

- 200 g of dried tomatoes
- ¼ pack every one of parsley and basil

- 3 teaspoons of capers
- 1 tbsp balsamic vinegar
- 150 ml of tomato oil
- 1 clove of garlic
- 100 g blended salad
- 500 g of bison mozzarella
- salt and pepper

Preparation:

1. First you put the tomatoes, alongside the washed spices and tricks, in a beaker.
2. Then you add the vinegar and tomato oil.
3. Everything is pounded into a smooth mass that you can prepare with salt and pepper.
4. Now you wash the plate of mixed greens and cut the mozzarella into slices.
5. The cheddar is partitioned on the plate of mixed greens and sprinkled with the tomato puree.

340 kcal/25g E/25g F/3g K

Mint flavored pea soup

A joy for the sense of taste and eyes.

20 minutes

Ingredients:

- 500 g peas, frozen
- 1 clove of garlic
- 2 shallots
- 1/2 lemon
- 1 liter of vegetable stock
- 150 g harsh cream
- 5 teaspoons of cleaved mint
- 5 teaspoons of hacked parsley
- 2 tbsp olive oil
- salt and pepper

Preparation:

1. Peel the garlic and shallots, cut them into fine 3D squares

and sauté them in a pot with a little oil until translucent.

2. Now you add the frozen peas and the lemon strip, pour everything with a liter of stock and allowed it to stew for around 8 minutes.

3. Then add half of the sharp cream to the soup and add the parsley and a big part of the mint.

4. Everything is presently finely pureed and, contingent upon your taste and the ideal consistency, weakened with a little broth.

5. The soup is then prepared with lemon squeeze, salt and pepper and decorated with a little acrid cream and a little mint.

200 kcal/10g E/10g F/17g K

Omelette with roasted mushrooms

If you like mushrooms, you will cherish their desire for mix with an omelette.

20 minutes

Ingredients:

- 8 eggs
- 200 g mushrooms
- 5 tbsp milk
- 2 teaspoons of turmeric paste
- 6 teaspoons of coriander
- 2 tbsp oil
- Paprika powder, honorable sweet
- salt and pepper

Preparation:

1. Clean the mushrooms and cut them into bits of equivalent size.

2. Then you put the eggs in a bowl and blend them in with the milk, the turmeric glue, 3 teaspoons of coriander, ½ teaspoon of paprika powder and 1 teaspoon of salt.

3. Then you put a few oil in a container and singe the mushrooms on all sides.

4. Then you pour the egg combination over it and fry everything over medium hotness for another three minutes.

5. Now you put the dish in the preheated broiler (200 °) and

let the omelet keep on cooking in the stove until it is set.
6. Finally, embellish it with the remainder of the

coriander. 245 kcal/17g E/19g F/1g K

Zoodles with pesto and cherry tomatoes

Low carb pasta is best produced using zucchinis. They look practically like genuine noodles and, as is notable, the eyes eat with them.

20 minutes

Ingredients:

- 600 g zucchini
- 150 g cherry tomatoes
- 1 pot of basil
- 1 clove of garlic
- 70 g ground parmesan cheese
- 70 ml of olive oil
- salt and pepper

Preparation:

1. First you wash the basil and pluck the leaves from the stems.
2. Then you strip the garlic and cut it into huge cubes.
3. Now put the basil, parmesan, garlic and olive oil in a bowl and puree everything finely.
4. Then you taste the pesto with salt and pepper.
5. Now you wash the zucchinis and cut them into a spaghetti shape with a twisting cutter.
6. The tomatoes are washed and cut in half.
7. Then blend the zucchini noodles in with the tomato parts and the pesto.
8. At the end everything is embellished with a little

basil. 260 kcal/7g E/23g F/5g K

Broccoli soup with coconut

Broccoli soup with an especially extraordinary aroma.

15 minutes

Ingredients:

- 2 broccoli
- 2 little onions
- 2 cloves of garlic
- 4 cups of water
- 2 lots of rocket
- 1 lemon
- 2 teaspoons of coconut oil
- Chili powder
- salt and pepper

Preparation:

1. Peel the onions and garlic, cleave both into fine shapes and fry the entire thing in a pot with coconut oil.
2. Then add the broccoli florets and let it burn for another 4 minutes.
3. Now stifle it with the water, add a few pepper, salt and stew and let everything stew over medium heat.
4. After around nine minutes, the broccoli is done and you can take the pot off the stove.
5. Now you add the rocket and hack everything with a hand blender until you get a smooth soup.
6. Finally, add the lemon juice.

130 kcal/5g E/8g F/14g K

Pizza with a vegetable base

One of our cherished dishes is the pizza with a vegetable base. With it you don't need to manage without the Italian exemplary notwithstanding the low carb diet.

20 minutes

Ingredients:

- 500 g cauliflower, generally grated
- 2 eggs
- 100 g of ground Gouda cheese
- 2 tomatoes

- tomato sauce
- ham or tuna
- 50 g pizza cheese
- salt and pepper

Preparation:
1. First you preheat the stove to 200 °.
2. Then line a baking sheet with material paper.
3. The ground cauliflower is blended in with the Gouda cheddar, eggs and somewhat salt and pepper and afterward spread the completed blend on the baking paper.
4. It is presently prepared for around 10 minutes.
5. Then you can sprinkle the base with pureed tomatoes, tomatoes, vegetables, fish or ham and cheddar, contingent upon your taste, and prepare everything again for 10 minutes.

193 kcal/16g E/12g F/4g K

Salad with beetroot, feta cheese and oranges

This salad isn't just a blowout as far as taste, it likewise carries a great deal of shading to your plate.

10 mins

Ingredients:

- 800 g beetroot
- 2 oranges
- 120 g of feta
- 4 stalks of mint
- 4 teaspoons of lime juice
- Chili flakes
- salt and pepper

Preparation:
1. First you strip the beetroot and the orange and cut both into slices.
2. Now place one orange and one beetroot cut then again on the plate until every one of the cuts are utilized up.
3. The feta cheddar is disintegrated over the cuts with

your hands.

4. Then sprinkle everything with the lime squeeze and sprinkle the mint and stew chips over it.

5. Finally, season everything with salt and pepper.

165 kcal/9g E/6g F/18g K

Halloumi on chickpea salad

Chickpea salad is very filling and tastes truly heavenly in mix with the halloumi.

20 minutes

Ingredients:

- 400 g of chickpeas
- 400 g halloumi
- 2 shallots
- 1 spring onion
- 60 g of radishes
- 100 g tomatoes
- 100 g paprika
- 100 g cucumber
- 40 g canned corn
- 4 teaspoons of slashed parsley
- 6 tbsp oil
- salt and pepper

Preparation:

1. First you put the chickpeas in a colander and flush them off with running water.

2. Then you heat a few oil in a container and fry the halloumi on the two sides and season it with somewhat salt and pepper.

3. Meanwhile, wash the vegetables and cut them into scaled down pieces.

4. The onions and shallots are additionally washed and cut into fine rings.

5. Then you put all the plate of mixed greens fixings in a bowl and mix them together well.

6. Then you add the olive oil and somewhat salt and

pepper and mix everything admirably again.

7. Finally, serve the serving of mixed greens along with the halloumi.

595 kcal/28g E/45g F/15g K

Colorful salad with spinach

This salad tastes extremely fascinating because of the mango and carries a totally different taste to the palate.

10 mins

Ingredients:

- 400 g of youthful spinach
- 500 g of mango
- 300 g paprika
- 60 g almonds
- 60 g of red onions
- 8 tbsp water
- 4 tbsp lime juice
- 2 tbsp apple juice vinegar
- some Xucker
- 4 stalks of coriander
- 1 bean stew pepper
- 2 cloves of garlic
- salt and pepper

Preparation:

1. First you strip the mangoes and cut the mash into cubes.
2. Then you wash the coriander, pluck the leaves and cleave them up.
3. The garlic is stripped and cut into 3D squares of the equivalent size.
4. The stew pepper is washed, divided and pitted.
5. Then you put 300 g of the mango mash along with the water, the lime squeeze, the apple juice vinegar, the xucker, the garlic and the bean stew in a bowl and puree everything with a blender until you get a fine dressing.
6. The dressing is currently prepared with salt and pepper and the coriander leaves are mixed in.
7. Now you wash the spinach leaves and eliminate the

stems.

8. The peppers are likewise washed, hollowed and cut into reduced down pieces.

9. Then you strip the onions and cut them into fine rings.

10. The almonds are generally chopped.

11. Now put the spinach, the remainder of the mango mash, the ringer pepper, the onion and the almonds in a bowl and blend every one of the fixings in with the dressing.

157 kcal/9g E/7g F/15g K

Salad with Swiss chard and feta

This salad tastes delightful, particularly in autumn.

10 mins

Ingredients:

- 200 g Swiss chard
- 200 g arugula
- 200 g youthful spinach
- 200 g feta cheese
- 200 g of dried tomatoes
- 4 tbsp hemp seeds
- 1 glass of dark olives
- 6 tbsp olive oil
- salt and pepper

Preparation:

1. First you wash the Swiss chard and rocket and twist everything dry.

2. Then you cut the feta into 3D shapes and blend it in with the sun-dried tomatoes, olives and hemp seeds.

3. Now you put the chard, spinach and rocket in an enormous bowl and blend everything with the feta mixture.

4. Finally, everything is showered with olive oil and prepared with somewhat salt and pepper.

350 kcal/19g E/24g F/13g K

Salad with fried pumpkin and Brussels sprouts

This formula is likewise especially appropriate for autumn.

20 minutes

Ingredients:

- 400 g of Hokkaido pumpkin
- 300 g Brussels sprouts
- 120 g pecans
- 40 g of cranberries
- 4 tbsp orange juice
- 2 tbsp olive oil
- salt and pepper

Preparation:

1. First, you wash the pumpkin and cut it into reduced down cubes.
2. Then you clean the Brussels fledglings and cut the florets in half.
3. Then you heat a few olive oil in a container and fry the Brussels fledglings and pumpkin on all sides.
4. Then you add the squeezed orange, the cranberries and the nuts and fry them as well.
5. Now you season everything with salt and pepper and mix it well again.

335 kcal/8g E/27g F/13g K

Side dishes

Spicy chanterelle pan

The chanterelle skillet is wonderful as a side dish for meat dishes. It gives the essential pep.

20 minutes

Ingredients:

- 1200 g of chanterelles
- 2 onions
- 2 cloves of garlic
- 2 tbsp butter

- 2 teaspoons of hacked rosemary
- 1 teaspoon cleaved thyme
- salt and pepper

Preparation:

1. First you clean the mushrooms. Then, at that point, you strip the onions and garlic and cut them into fine cubes.
2. Then put a few spread and oil in a dish and fry the garlic and onions in it.
3. Then add the rosemary and thyme and mix all that well.
4. Then add the mushrooms to the container and singe them until they are somewhat brown.
5. Meanwhile you taste everything with salt and

pepper. 240 kcal/10g E/20g F/5g K

Avocado in a bacon costume

Not just dates taste especially zesty enclosed by bacon. You ought to likewise attempt avocados.

20 minutes

Ingredients:

- 4 avocados
- juice of a lime
- 600 grams of bacon
- 2 tbsp olive oil
- salt and pepper

Preparation:

1. First you cut the avocados down the middle and eliminate the stones.
2. Then you cut it into quarters and eliminate the mash from

the skin.

3. Now you shower it with the lime squeeze so the bits of organic product don't discolour.
4. The bacon cuts are fanned out so you can move up the

avocado pieces in them.

5. Then you heat a few oil in a skillet and singe the avocados in bacon on all sides.

6. Finally, they are prepared with salt and pepper and served immediately.

450 kcal/14g E/42g F/2g K

Salad with arugula and cherry tomatoes

This salad tastes new in summer and goes similarly as with fish.

20 minutes

Ingredients:

- 400 g of rocket
- 400 g of cherry tomatoes
- 2 teaspoons of balsamic vinegar
- a hint of lemon juice
- 2 tbsp oil
- some nutmeg
- salt and pepper

Preparation:

1. First you wash the rocket and cut it into reduced down pieces.

2. Then you wash the tomatoes and cut them in half.

3. Now put the balsamic cream with the olive oil, lemon juice, nutmeg, salt and pepper in a bowl and combine everything as one well.

4. Finally, blend the rocket in with the tomatoes and enhancement everything with the dressing.

83 kcal/4g E/5g F/5g K

Eggplant fries

French fries don't continuously need to be produced using potatoes or yams. They likewise get their appeal from eggplants.

20 minutes

Ingredients:

- 520 g almond flour

- 4 eggplants
- 4 eggs
- olive oil
- Paprika powder, honorable sweet
- garlic powder
- salt and pepper

Preparation:

1. First you strip the eggplants and cut them into french fries.
2. Then you put the eggs in a plate and whisk them together.
3. The almond flour is blended in a moment plate with the paprika powder, the garlic powder and the pepper.
4. Now you take the fries and turn them first in the beaten egg and afterward in the almond mixture.
5. The fries are then prepared in a preheated broiler (200 °) for around 5 minutes.
6. Then they are brushed with a little olive oil and heated for an additional ten minutes until they are crispy.

540 kcal/32g E/43g F/6g K

Mushroom pan with fennel

This mushroom skillet additionally goes impeccably with meat dishes.

20 minutes

Ingredients:

- 800 g mushrooms
- 300 g of fennel
- Two lemons
- 2 teaspoons of slashed rosemary
- 4 cloves of garlic
- 2 teaspoons of ground ginger
- 4 tbsp oil
- 2 tbsp butter
- 2 straight leaves
- some nutmeg
- salt and pepper

Preparation:

1. First, you clean the mushrooms, eliminate the stems and cut them into slices.
2. Then you clean the fennel and cut it into cuts as well.
3. The garlic is additionally stripped and cut into fine slices.
4. Then you heat a few margarine and oil in a container and fry the garlic until brilliant brown.
5. Now you add the mushrooms and the fennel and keep on searing everything.
6. Meanwhile, pour a few lemon juice and the ginger over it and mix all that well.
7. Then add the rosemary and cove passes on and keep on fricasseeing everything for a couple minutes.
8. Finally, taste everything with a little nutmeg and pepper. 169 kcal/7g E/14g F/4g K

Zucchini - mushroom - pan

An ideal side dish for a grill evening.

20 minutes

Ingredients:

- 1000 g mushrooms
- 2 zucchini
- 2 stew peppers
- 4 shallots
- 1 bundle of parsley, chopped
- 1 piece of ginger
- some nutmeg
- 2 tbsp olive oil
- salt and pepper

Preparation:

1. Clean the mushrooms and zucchini and cut both into dainty slices.
2. Then you wash the stew, eliminate the seeds and cut them into meager cuts as well.
3. The shallots and ginger are likewise stripped and cut into fine cubes.

4. Now you heat some oil in a container and momentarily fry the shallots, mushrooms and zucchini.

5. The stew and ginger are additionally added and everything is singed until the mushrooms and zucchini are cooked through.

6. Finally, taste everything with nutmeg, salt and pepper and appreciate it with the new parsley.

150 kcal/15g E/7g F/8g K

Tomato salsa

Suitable as a side dish for practically any meat.

20 minutes

Ingredients:

- 500 g tomatoes
- 1 red pepper
- 1 stew pepper
- 1 onion
- 2 cloves of garlic
- ½ lime
- 1 tbsp hacked parsley
- 4 tablespoons of olive oil
- 1 tbsp balsamic vinegar, white
- 1 spot of Xucker
- salt and pepper

Preparation:

1. Wash the tomatoes and cut them into cubes.

2. Then you strip the onion and the garlic and cut them into fine 3D shapes as well.

3. The peppers are additionally washed and diced.

4. Now put the tomatoes in a bowl and blend them in with the onions, garlic and peppers.

5. The parsley is likewise blended in.

6. Then you blend the olive oil in with the balsamic vinegar, salt and pepper in a cup until you get a vinaigrette.

7. The vinaigrette is then poured over the

salsa. 30 kcal/1g E/2g F/1g K

Baked fennel with a cheese topping

If you like fennel, you ought to attempt the blend with cheddar.

20 minutes

Ingredients:

- 1 kg of fennel
- 150 ml of cream
- 40 g butter
- ½ stew, chopped
- 50 g olives, chopped
- 125 g cheddar, grated
- salt

Preparation:

1. First you wash the fennel, slash the greens and cut the rest into quarters.

2. Then you cook the fennel in bubbling salted water for around 8 minutes.

3. Meanwhile you let the margarine dissolve in a baking dish, add the completed fennel quarters and pour the cream over it.

4. The olives and stew are likewise sprinkled on top and afterward covered with the ground cheddar.

5. Finally, everything needs to cook for around 10 minutes in the preheated stove (180 ° C) and is then decorated with the cleaved fennel greens.

420 kcal/16g E/34g F/8g K

Quick cucumber salad

Cucumber salad not just preferences very reviving, it additionally contains a great deal of water, which is significant for a sound diet.

5 minutes

Ingredients:

- 800 g cucumber
- 2 spring onions
- 2 teaspoons parsley, chopped
- 4 tablespoons of olive oil
- salt and pepper

Preparation:

1. First you wash the cucumber and cut it into slim slices.
2. Then you clean the spring onion and cut it into fine rings.
3. Then put the cucumber, onion and parsley in a bowl and blend them in with the olive oil.
4. Finally, everything is prepared with salt and pepper.

125 kcal/2g E/9g F/9g K

Mediterranean-style vegetables

This vegetable blend tastes incredible both as a fundamental course and as a side dish.

20 minutes

Ingredients:

- 2 zucchini
- 2 eggplants
- 2 peppers
- 2 onions
- 2 cloves of garlic
- 250 g mozzarella
- 100 g dark olives
- 4 tablespoons of olive oil
- 12 tbsp vegetable broth
- 2 teaspoons of rosemary, chopped
- salt and pepper

Preparation:

1. First you wash the eggplant, zucchini, and peppers.
2. The eggplant and zucchini are cut into cuts and the peppers into cubes.
3. Now you strip the garlic and the onions and cut them into fine 3D shapes as well.

4. Then you heat a few olive oil in a container and fry the diced paprika and the vegetable cuts in it.
5. Then you add the onion, garlic and rosemary and keep on browning for a couple minutes.
6. Then you erase everything with the vegetable stock and let it stew briefly.
7. Meanwhile, cut the mozzarella into 3D squares and blend it in with somewhat olive oil.
8. The vegetables are put in a bowl and blended in with the mozzarella mixture.
9. Finally, everything is prepared with salt and pepper.

220 kcal/8g E/15g F/7g K

Cauliflower croquettes

Croquettes don't constantly need to be potatoes. They taste tasty even from cauliflower.

20 minutes

Ingredients:

- 500 g of cauliflower
- 400 g coconut oil
- 120 g almonds
- 20g of potato fibers
- 20g coconut flour
- 3 tablespoons of carob gum
- 3 eggs
- 1 teaspoon vegetable stock powder
- 2 tbsp parsley, chopped

Preparation:

1. First you clean the cauliflower and relax the florets.
2. They are then bubbled in a pan of bubbling salted water for around 7 minutes.
3. Then you pour off the water and puree the cauliflower until it turns into a pulp.
4. Now you separate the eggs and add the yolks to the puree. The egg white is put on a plate for the time being.
5. Now you add the parsley, the vegetable powder, the potato filaments, the insect bean gum and salt and pepper to

the cauliflower and blend everything together.

6. Then you take a plate and mix the almonds and coconut flour on it.

7. The puree is presently framed into little balls and turned in a steady progression in the egg white and in the almond mixture.

8. Then you heat the coconut oil in a huge container and add the croquettes.

9. They are seared firm brown on all sides. 235 kcal/8g E/20g F/5g K

Creamy carrot soup with soured milk

This soup is exceptionally famous with us, particularly on the chilly days, and we regularly eat it in the evening so we are easily warm.

15 minutes

Ingredients:

- 500 g of carrots
- 500 ml of meat broth
- 250 ml of milk
- 180 ml of curd milk
- 1 tbsp parsley, chopped
- salt and pepper

Preparation:

1. First you clean the carrots and cut them into fine slices.
2. Then you heat half of the stock to the point of boiling and cook the carrots in it.
3. Then you puree everything and set it back in the pot.
4. Now you add the remainder of the stock, the milk and the curd and let everything boil.
5. The soup is then prepared with salt and pepper and, in the wake of parceling, decorated with the parsley.

125 kcal/9g E/6g F/8g K

Cottage cheese salad

Cheese is especially wealthy in protein and low in starches and is thusly entirely appropriate for a low carb diet.

5 minutes

Ingredients:

- 800 g of bungalow cheese
- 500 g of celery
- 4 tbsp basil
- 8 tbsp linseed oil
- 4 tbsp lemon juice
- salt and pepper

Preparation:

1. First you strip the celery and mesh it into huge pieces.
2. Then you blend the curds with the celery and the basil in a bowl.
3. Everything is prepared with salt and pepper.
4. Finally, add the linseed oil and lemon juice. 198 kcal/12g E/14g F/4g K

Parsley root fries

These fries have an exceptionally extraordinary taste and are a welcome change.

20 minutes

Ingredients:

- 600 g parsley root
- 2 cloves of garlic
- 2 teaspoons of Provence herbs
- 1 teaspoon salt
- 20 tbsp olive oil

Preparation:

1. First you strip the parsley roots and cut them into french fries.
2. Then you strip the garlic and press it out.
3. Now you mix the oil, spices, garlic and salt into a marinade.
4. Then the fries are marinated with it and put close to one another on a baking sheet with baking paper.

5. Finally, the fries are prepared in a preheated broiler (180 ° C) for around 15 minutes until they are crispy.

350 kcal/5g E/32g F/10g K

Sweets and cakes

Basic recipe for chia pudding

This pudding is wealthy in protein and filling, making it a decent substitute for ordinary pudding.

5 minutes

Ingredients:

- 4 tbsp chia seeds
- 250 ml almond milk, unsweetened
- some new vanilla

Preparation:

1. First you put the chia seeds, the almond milk and the vanilla in a bowl and combine everything as one well.
2. Then you let the pudding drench for the time being and you can increase it or simply eat it, contingent upon your taste.

270 kcal/14g E/21g F/4g K

Fresh low carb waffles

Waffles are extremely famous, particularly in the virus season. In the low carb variation, they actually fit into the sustenance plan.

20 minutes

Ingredients:

- 80g butter
- 3 eggs
- 1 ½ tsp stevia
- 80g almonds (ground)
- ½ tsp baking powder
- 1 banana
- 500ml whipped cream

- 1 smidgen of orange juice

Preparation:

1. Mash the banana with a fork and beat it along with the spread and eggs until frothy.
2. In a different bowl, blend the xylitol, baking powder and ground almonds.
3. Mix the substance of the two dishes cautiously into a homogeneous batter.
4. Grease your waffle iron and prepare your waffles in it.
5. Beat the whipped cream along with a hint of squeezed orange until firm and embellishment your waffles with it

273 kcal/5.2g E/23.3g F/8.5g K (with 10 servings)

nut cookies

With these treats, those with a sweet tooth who eat as indicated by the low carb standard will get their cash's worth.

20 minutes

Ingredients:

- 4 tbsp almonds, chopped
- 4 tbsp cashew nuts, chopped
- 4 sans stone dates, chopped
- 2 egg yolks
- 150 g of ground almonds
- 60 g butter
- Some Xucker

Preparation:

1. First you put the margarine in a pot and let it dissolve over low heat.
2. Then you blend the margarine in a bowl in with the almonds, cashew nuts and dates and mix in the eggs, flour and xucker.
3. From the completed mixture, 24 little balls are currently shaped, which you then, at that point, smooth into thalers on a baking sheet with baking paper.
4. The rolls are then heated in a preheated broiler (180 ° C)

for around 10 minutes.

78 kcal/3g E/7g F/2g K (per biscuit)

Low carb crepes with berry filling

These crepes are not just heavenly; the berries additionally give them a fruity freshness.

20 minutes

Ingredients:

- 100 g spelled flour
- 100 g almond flour
- 30 g coconut flour
- 2 eggs
- 300 ml of water
- salt
- 8 tbsp normal yogurt
- 80 g blended berries
- some Xucker

Preparation:

1. First you put the flour, eggs, salt and water in a bowl and combine everything as one well.
2. Then put the batter in segments (4) in a covered container and heat it well on both sides.
3. When the crepes have chilled off a little, cover them with the yogurt and pour the berries over them.
4. Then you crease the crêpes together and, contingent upon your taste, sprinkle them with a little Xucker.

290 kcal/20g E/10g F/27g K

Hot drinking chocolate

The hot cocoa warms you on cool days and helps promptly when you want something sweet.

12 minutes

Ingredients:

- 800 ml coconut milk
- 400 ml of water
- 200 ml of cream
- 2 teaspoons of cinnamon
- 1 vanilla pod
- 2 tbsp xylitol
- 6 tbsp cocoa, sugar-free
- some salt

Preparation:

1. First you heat the coconut milk in a saucepan.
2. Meanwhile, add the vanilla, cinnamon, xylitol, cocoa and salt and mix everything well.
3. Then you mix in the water.
4. Finally, whip the cream until solid and disperse it over all the portions.

450 kcal/8g E/41g F/9g K

marzipan potatoes

What might the Christmas prepare be without marzipan potatoes? Luckily, there is additionally a low-carb variant of these little treats.

14 minutes

Ingredients:

- 100 g of ground almonds
- 80 g powder xucker
- 7 drops of severe almond flavor
- 2 tbsp cocoa, sugar-free
- 1 tbsp coconut oil
- 2 tbsp water

Preparation:

1. First you put the ground almonds in a bowl and blend them in with the powder xucker.
2. Then you steadily work in the coconut oil, the water and the almond flavor.
3. Now you manipulate everything until the mixture is

moldable and marginally sticky.

4. Then you structure little balls out of the batter, which you then, at that point, just turn in a bowl with cocoa.

45 kcal/1g E/4g F/1g K (per scoop)

chocolate pudding

A chocolate pudding not just causes you to feel full; it likewise satisfies you. With this formula variation, it likewise squeezes into your low carb menu.

15 minutes

Ingredients:

- 200 ml of water
- 100 ml of cream
- 50 g cocoa, sugar-free
- 3 teaspoons of erythritol
- 3 egg yolks
- 1 teaspoon carob flour
- 4 teaspoons of raspberries

Preparation:

1. First you heat up the water and add the cream and cocoa.
2. Then you taste the pudding with erythritol.
3. Then you mix the egg yolks and the carob gum in a bowl to a homogeneous mass.
4. Now you mix the egg yolk combination into the pudding.
5. After a couple of moments of mixing, the pudding ought to get the ideal consistency.
6. All parts are embellished with the new raspberries.

180 kcal/6g E/15g F/5g K

Breakfast and bread

Scrambled eggs with chorizo pieces

The proper thing for each and every individual who likes it generous in the morning.

20 minutes

Ingredients:

- 1 red pepper
- 2 spring onions
- 150 g chorizo sausage
- 6 eggs
- 4 tbsp milk
- 1 tbsp olive oil
- salt and pepper

Preparation:

1. Wash the peppers and leeks and cut both into little pieces.
2. The wiener is likewise cut into equally estimated pieces and afterward momentarily burned on all sides in a container with blistering oil.
3. Then add the peppers and onions and fry them briefly.
4. Meanwhile, whisk the eggs with the milk and season the blend with salt and pepper.
5. Then you add the egg combination to the skillet and let the egg set while you blend everything together.

340 kcal/21g E/26g F/4g K

Omelette with cheese and peppers

An especially hot omelette.

15 minutes

Ingredients:

- 250 g youthful spinach leaves
- 1 little onion
- 1 clove of garlic
- 3 tbsp oil
- 60 g parmesan cheddar, grated
- 8 eggs
- 200 g paprika curd
- Salt and pepper and nutmeg

Preparation:

1. Peel the onion and garlic, cut them into fine shapes, wash and channel the spinach.
2. Fry the onion and garlic in a little oil, add the spinach and let it collapse.
3. Season everything with nutmeg, salt and pepper, separate the eggs and beat the egg whites until stiff.
4. Then blend the egg yolks in with the parmesan and spinach and crease in the egg white.
5. Everything is singed in a dish with a little oil and afterward prepared in a preheated broiler (200 ° C) for another 10 minutes.
6. Season the quark with a little pepper and serve it with the omelette.

395 kcal/27g E/30g F/3g K

Omelette with goat cheese and nuts

The goat cheddar gives this omelet an extremely hot aroma.

20 minutes

Ingredients:

- 2 red onions
- 1/2 bundle of spring onions
- 200 g delicate goat cheese
- 8 eggs
- 5 tbsp whipped cream
- 50 g pecan kernels
- 3 teaspoons of oil
- some Xucker
- salt and pepper

Preparation:

1. Peel the onions and leeks, cut everything into fine rings and gap the goat cheddar into 8 slices.
2. Whisk the eggs with the cream and salt and pepper and toast the pecans in a non-oiled pan.
3. Then you heat a few oil and singe the onions and leeks.
4. Put ¼ of the egg combination in a dish and let the egg set

with the top closed.

    5. The completed omelet is finished off with ¼ of the onion blend and 2 cuts of goat cheddar and afterward closed.

    6. Then rehash all that multiple times until you have completed 4 servings and embellishment them with simmered nuts.

$$520 \text{ kcal}/28g \text{ E}/41g \text{ F}/7g \text{ K}$$

Scrambled chocolate eggs

An uncommon formula. In any case, the outcome is convincing.

15 minutes

Ingredients:

- 12 eggs
- 60 g almond butter
- 4 teaspoons of erythritol
- 20 g coconut oil
- 60 g without sugar chocolate drops
- 600 g of product of your choice

Preparation:

    1. Whisk the eggs with the erythritol and almond butter.
    2. Fry them in a non-leave dish with a little coconut oil, blending occasionally.
    3. As soon as the egg is set, add the chocolate drops.
    4. Garnish with your fruit.

$$421 \text{ kcal}/21g \text{ E}/29g \text{ F}/15.5g \text{ K}$$

Carrot drink with oranges

This blend of vegetables and natural products brings about a flavorful and empowering drink.

5 minutes

Ingredients:

- 4 oranges
- 4 carrots

- 200 g apples
- 4 g ginger, grated
- 4 portions of cinnamon
- 400 ml of cold water

Preparation:

1. First you crush the oranges.
2. Then you clean the carrots and cut them into pieces.
3. Then you cut the apples into pieces and eliminate the stones.
4. Then, at that point, you put every one of the fixings in the blender and puree them into a smoothie.

117 kcal/2g E/0g F/27g K

Fried egg with bacon

If you want a good breakfast, you ought to attempt this recipe.

10 mins

Ingredients:

- 8 eggs
- 120 g breakfast bacon
- 8 tbsp olive oil
- salt and pepper

Preparation:

1. First you heat a few oil in a container and fry the morning meal bacon in it until crispy.
2. Then you shove the bacon to the aside and break the eggs in the pan.
3. They are singed over medium hotness and prepared with salt and pepper.
4. The eggs are then presented with the

bacon. 405 kcal/18g E/36g F/2g K

Low carb porridge with coconut

The porridge with coconut flour tastes extraordinary and is normally improved by the vanilla.

10 mins

Ingredients:

- 800 ml of water
- 100 ml of cream
- 150 g coconut flour
- 1 vanilla pod
- 50 g parched coconut
- 2 eggs
- some Xucker

Preparation:

1. First you divide the vanilla unit lengthways and scratch it out.
2. Then you heat the cream and water in a pot and add the vanilla, coconut flour and dried up coconut.
3. Everything must now cook for around 5 minutes, stirring constantly.
4. Then you take the pot off the oven and mix the egg into the porridge with a whisk.
5. Everything is then briefly heated again and finally prepared with a little Xucker.

460 kcal/28g E/36g F/5g K

Low carb porridge with almonds and flax seeds

With porridge you can fulfill your craving in a flavorful manner for a long time.

20 minutes

Ingredients:

- 400 ml of coconut milk
- 400 ml of water
- 8 tbsp squashed flaxseed
- 120 g ground almonds
- 2 tbsp chia seeds
- Xucker

Preparation:

1. First you heat the coconut milk and the water in a saucepan.
2. Then you add the flax seeds, the ground almonds, the chia seeds and the salt and let everything stew for around 8 minutes. You should mix occasionally.
3. Finally, you can improve the porridge with

Xucker. 420 kcal/22g E/34g F/5g K

Cinnamon-flavored banana muffins

These sweet biscuits are ensured to fulfill your sweet tooth.

20 minutes

Ingredients:

- 240 g protein powder (vanilla)
- 8 eggs
- 8 bananas
- 8 teaspoons of baking powder
- 8 teaspoons of cinnamon powder
- 16 tbsp low-fat quark
- 8 portions of salt
- 16 tbsp nuts, chopped

Preparation:

1. First you pound the bananas with a fork and whisk them with the eggs and low-fat quark.
2. Then add the egg white powder, baking powder, cinnamon and salt and combine everything as one well.
3. Now mix in the nuts too.
4. Then you put the mixture in a biscuit skillet and prepare the biscuits in the preheated broiler (175 ° C) for around 12 minutes.

395 kcal/32g E/20g F/18g K

25 bonus recipes for on the go

Greek style salad

This salad is amazing to take away.

15 minutes

Ingredients:

- 1 head of lettuce
- 1 little cucumber
- 1 tomato
- 1 onion
- 2 cloves of garlic
  - 350 g artichoke hearts (glass)
  - 75 g of sheep cheese
  - 5 tbsp yogurt dressing
  - 1 tbsp oregano (dried)

Preparation:

1. Wash the lettuce, tomatoes, and cucumber and cut everything into reduced down pieces.
2. Then you strip the onion and cut it into fine rings. The garlic is likewise stripped and finely chopped.
3. Now you disintegrate the sheep's cheddar and let the artichoke hearts trickle off.
4. Now combine every one of the fixings as one and pour the dressing and oregano over the plate of mixed greens before consumption.

145 kcal/11g E/4.3g F/12g K

Cucumber salad with chopped mint

This salad gets an exceptionally extraordinary smell on the off chance that you let it steep for the time being. So it tastes great the following day.

20 minutes

Ingredients:

- 2 cucumbers
- ½ pack of new mint, chopped
- 4 tbsp safflower oil
- 1 tbsp white wine vinegar

- 1 tbsp orange juice
- 1 teaspoon of orange bloom water
- salt and pepper

Preparation:

1. First you eliminate the skin of the cucumber and cut it into fine slices.
2. Then you blend them in a bowl in with the slashed mint leaves.
3. Now you put the vinegar, the oil, the squeezed orange, the orange bloom water, salt and pepper in a bowl and combine everything as one well.
4. Then you pour the dressing over the plate of mixed greens, combine everything as one well and let it splash through.

96 kcal/1g E/9g F/1.7g K

Fruity salad with pomegranate and quail eggs

The pomegranate seeds and the quail eggs add a unique flavor to this recipe.

10 mins

Ingredients:

- 400 g sheep's lettuce
- 200 g cherry tomatoes
- 16 dark olives, pitted
- 12 quail eggs
- 120 g pomegranate seeds
- 4 tablespoons of olive oil
- 4 teaspoons of sesame seeds
- salt and pepper

Preparation:

1. First you heat up the quail eggs hard in steaming hot water for 4 minutes.
2. Then you wash the lettuce and channel the olives.
3. Then wash the tomatoes and cut them in half.
4. Now you put the sheep's lettuce in a bowl and blend it

in with the olives, tomatoes and pomegranate seeds.

5. Then you pour the oil over the salad and season everything with salt and pepper.

6. Finally, pellet and divide the eggs and add them to the plate of mixed greens along with the sesame seeds.

305 kcal/10g E/24g F/11g K

Mushrooms with cream cheese filling

A truly fine taste experience.

20 minutes

Ingredients:

- 1 kg of mushrooms
- 300 g of cream cheese
- 2 lemons
- 4 spring onions
- 200 g parmesan, grated
- 4 tablespoons of olive oil
- 2 cloves of garlic
- 2 teaspoons parsley, chopped
- nutmeg
- salt and pepper

Preparation:

1. Clean the mushrooms, eliminate the stems, hack them, and put them on a baking sheet fixed with material paper.

2. Peel the onions and garlic, cut both into little pieces and mesh the lemon peel.

3. Fry the onions, garlic and mushroom follows momentarily and add the cream cheddar and lemon zing. Season everything with nutmeg, salt and pepper.

4. The completed the process of filling then, at that point, goes into the mushrooms and everything is sprinkled with the parmesan.

5. The filled mushrooms should now be heated in the preheated broiler (200 ° C) for around 12 minutes and decorated with the parsley for serving.

615 kcal/37g E/49g F/3g K

Broccoli salad with quinoa

Quinoa isn't just wealthy in protein, yet additionally an extraordinary filling side dish.

- 400 g broccoli
- 200 grams of quinoa
- 150 g paprika
- 12 cherry tomatoes
- 80 g of rocket
- 4 tbsp lime juice
- 4 tablespoons of olive oil
- salt and pepper

20 minutes
Ingredients:

Preparation:
1. First you wash the quinoa off under running water.
2. Then you let them bubble in a pot of water for around 8 minutes.
3. Meanwhile, wash the broccoli florets and bubble them in steaming hot water for around 5 minutes until they are firm to the bite.
4. After cooking, the quinoa is prepared with salt, pepper and lime juice.
5. Now you wash the peppers, tomatoes and rocket and cut everything into reduced down pieces.
6. Finally, layer every one of the vegetables on the other hand in a glass and shower the bits with a little oil.

300 kcal/13g E/12g F/34g K

Paprika with cheese filling

This light dish rushes to make, yet in addition exceptionally delectable the following day when chilled.

10 mins

Ingredients:

- 2 red peppers
- 400 g of bungalow cheese
- 200 g of radishes
- 2 tbsp chives, chopped
- salt and pepper

Preparation:

1. First you wash the peppers, cut them down the middle and eliminate the seeds.
2. Then you wash the radishes and cut them into slight slices.
3. Now put the cream cheddar and the curds in a bowl and blend them in with the radishes and chives.
4. The mass is then prepared with salt and pepper.
5. Finally, empty the combination into the pepper parts and serve.

134 kcal/14g E/5g F/8g K

Tomatoes with ricotta filling

As a filling for our tomatoes, ricotta is a hit at our family table.

20 minutes

Ingredients:

- 4 enormous tomatoes
- 40 g green olives, pitted
- 4 radishes
- 1 spring onion
- 100 g ricotta
- 100 g of cream cheese
- 2 teaspoons of basil, chopped
- cress
- Salt and pepper and nutmeg

Preparation:

1. First, you wash the tomatoes, remove the top cover, and eliminate the seeds with a spoon.
2. Clean the radishes and cut them into fine cubes.
3. Then you slash the olives and cut the onion into fine rings.
4. Now you put the cream cheddar in a bowl and blend it in with the ricotta, olives, basil, radishes and onions.
5. The combination is prepared with salt, pepper and nutmeg and filled the tomatoes.
6. Finally, embellish every one of the segments

with a little cress. 140 kcal/5g E/11g F/5g K

Asian broccoli salad

If you like it outlandish, you ought to attempt this salad.

20 minutes

Ingredients:

- 800 grams of broccoli
- 4 carrots
- 2 tomatoes
- 400 ml of warm water
- 100 ml soy sauce
- 4 tbsp sesame oil
- 2 teaspoons of sesame seeds
- some Xucker
- salt and pepper

Preparation:

1. Wash the broccoli florets and tomatoes and cut them into reduced down pieces.
2. Then you clean the carrots and cut them into slices.
3. Heat the sesame oil in a container and fry the broccoli and carrots well on all sides.
4. Then you add the tomatoes and season everything great with salt and pepper.
5. The soy sauce is blended in with the water and the xucker in a bowl and furthermore added to the pan.
6. Everything must now stew for a couple minutes.
7. Finally, season the serving of mixed greens with salt and pepper again and

decorate with the sesame seeds.

220 kcal/12g E/13g F/13g K

Gazpacho soup

Even heated up is a genuine joy and is consequently great for the office.

20 minutes

Ingredients:

- 800g ready tomatoes
- 2 red onions
- 6 cloves of garlic
- 2 green peppers
- 2 stewed cucumbers
- basil leaves
- 2 tablespoons of wine vinegar
- 4 tablespoons of olive oil
- salt and pepper

Preparation:

1. First you strip the tomatoes, center them and cut them into quarters. Presently strip the onion and garlic.
2. The cucumbers are additionally stripped, cut down the middle and pitted.
3. Now you center the peppers and cut them into strips.
4. Now you take 1/3 of the vegetables and cut them into blocks of the equivalent size.
5. The leftover vegetables are pureed along with the oil and vinegar and prepared with salt and pepper.
6. Then you blend the vegetables in with the soup and topping everything with a couple of basil leaves.

155 kcal/2g E/10g F/13g K

Fast fruit salad "to go"

This natural product salad tastes sweet and is extraordinary as a nibble for the office.

10 mins

Ingredients:

- 4 pears
- Kernels of 2 pomegranates
- 80 g pecans, chopped

Preparation:

1. First you wash the pear, eliminate the stones and cut it

into flimsy slices.
2. Then you put some pear cuts in a glass first.
3. Then layer the pomegranate seeds and nuts on top.
4. You do this until every one of the fixings are

spent. 220 kcal/4g E/14g F/18g K

Juicy chicken breast with a side salad

This dish is great for the workplace since you can get ready everything rapidly and effectively at home.

20 minutes

Ingredients:

- 500 g of chicken breast
- 200 g tomatoes
- 120 g rocket
- 40 g pine nuts
- 5 tbsp olive oil
- salt and pepper

Preparation:

1. First you wash the rocket and tomatoes and cut everything into reduced down pieces.
2. Then brown the pine nuts in a skillet without oil and blend them in with the tomatoes and rocket to make a salad.
3. Then you wash the chicken and fry it on all sides in a pan with hot oil.
4. Then you season it with salt and pepper and orchestrate it with the salad.

470 kcal/35g E/34g F/4g K

Vegetarian steaks with tomato salad

This formula comes without meat and still guarantees full enjoyment.

20 minutes

Ingredients:

- 1 kg of cauliflower
- 400 g tomatoes
- 2 eggs
- 200 g Gouda cheddar, grated
- 1 teaspoon dill, chopped
- 1 teaspoon parsley, chopped
- 4 tablespoons of olive oil
- Salt and pepper and nutmeg

Preparation:

1. First, you wash the cauliflower and rub it with the grater until it has a semolina-like consistency.
2. Then you put the cauliflower, along with the eggs, the Gouda, the nutmeg, salt and pepper in a bowl and blend everything into a batter.
3. The tomatoes are washed, cut into cuts and appropriated on the plates.
4. Then you season them with salt and pepper and enhancement with the herbs.
5. Then you heat some oil in a container, shape the mixture into uniformly estimated flatbreads and fry them until brilliant brown on both sides.
6. Finally, add the steaks to the tomato salad.

390 kcal/22g E/28g F/9g K

- 4 eggs

Cloud bread

Light and breezy low carb rolls 10 mins

Ingredients:

- 100g cream cheddar (0.2% fat)

Preparation:

1. Separate the yolks from the egg white.
2. Mix the egg yolks with the cream cheddar and beat the egg whites very stiff.
3. Carefully lift the egg whites into the cream cheddar combination and line a baking sheet with material paper.
4. Form little mists out of the batter and prepare them at 160 °C until they are firm and a little brownish.

86 kcal/8.3g E/1.6g F/5g K

Cherry yoghurt with an exotic coconut filling

The coconut filling gives this yogurt an extremely extraordinary bite.

10 mins

Ingredients:

- 800 g of yogurt
- 400 g of new cherries
- 40 g cocoa nibs
- 40 g almonds
- 80 g coconut chips
- some Xucker

Preparation:

1. First, you wash the cherries, stone them, and cut them in half.
2. Then you put the cherries, along with the yogurt, in a bowl and puree all that finely.
3. Then blend the hacked almonds in with the cocoa chips and cocoa nibs and pour the blend over all the portions.

452 kcal/14g E/30g F/29g K

Cherry smoothie

You can likewise invoke a sound and delectable smoothie from cherries.

5 minutes

Ingredients:

- 400 g cherries, pitted
- 2 little apples
- 800 ml of cold water

Preparation:

1. First, you wash the cherries, stone them, and cut them in half.
2. Then you wash the apples, center them and cut them into bits of the equivalent size.
3. The cherries and apples are presently positioned in a mug alongside the water and pounded into a smoothie.

90 kcal/1g E/0g F/21g K

Red cabbage salad with apples

The kinds of apple and red cabbage not just go magnificently along with the Christmas duck.

10 mins

Ingredients:

- 400 g red cabbage
- 12 radishes
- 120 g apples
- 80 g of red onions
- 4 teaspoons of coriander, chopped
- 8 tbsp olive oil
- some Xucker
- 4 teaspoons of sesame seeds
- 4 smidgens of lime juice
- salt

Preparation:

1. First you clean the red cabbage and cut it into fine strips.

Then, at that point, you strip the onions and cut them into fine strips.

2. The radishes and apples are additionally cut into fine slices.
3. Then you orchestrate the red cabbage, alongside the onions, apples and radishes.
4. The oil is blended in a bowl with the lime juice, coriander and xucker to make a dressing and sprinkled over the salad.

276 kcal/3g E/21g F/18g K

Low carb porridge with nuts

This porridge will keep you full for quite a while and, gratitude to the nuts, gives important oils to your health.

10 mins

Ingredients:

- 800 ml almond milk
- 100 g pecan parts, ground
- 80 g flaxseed, crushed
- 40 g of oatmeal
- some Xucker
- 2 teaspoons of cinnamon
- 4 portions of salt
- 200 g of raspberries
- 200 g blueberries

Preparation:

1. First you heat the milk in a little saucepan.
2. Then you add the pecans, the flax seeds and the oat pieces and mix everything well.
3. Cinnamon and salt are likewise added and afterward stewed for around 6 minutes.
4. Depending on your taste, you can improve the porridge with the Xucker.
5. Finally, decorate the segments with the

berries. 355 kcal/12g E/27g F/14g K

Quick tomato salad

Tomato salad isn't just sound, however for this situation it rushes to make.

5 minutes

Ingredients:

- 800 g tomatoes
- 2 teaspoons parsley, chopped
- 2 teaspoons of basil, chopped
- 4 tbsp balsamic vinegar
- salt and pepper

Preparation:

1. First you wash the tomatoes and cut them into blocks of the equivalent size.
2. Then you season them with salt and pepper.
3. Finally, add the parsley, basil and balsamic vinegar. 62 kcal/2g E/0g F/13g K

zucchini soup

This soup is filling and simple to process. It is accordingly ideal for the lunch break.

- 800 g zucchini
- 2 onions
- 2 cloves of garlic
- 100 g of potatoes

20 minutes

Ingredients:

- 1 teaspoon thyme, chopped
- 1 teaspoon rosemary, chopped
- 1 l vegetable stock
- 200 ml of cream
- 8 tbsp olive oil
- 2 tbsp butter
- nutmeg
- salt and pepper

Preparation:

1. First you wash the zucchini and cut them into 3D squares of the equivalent size.
2. Then you strip the garlic and onions and cut them into fine cubes.
3. The potatoes are additionally stripped and generally grated.
4. Now you put a few margarine and oil in a pot and fry the onions and garlic in it.
5. Then you add the potatoes and steam them with.
6. Then erase everything with the stock and let it stew for around 7 minutes with the top closed.
7. Then you likewise add the zucchini and let everything stew for another 5 minutes.
8. Finally, take the soup off the oven and mix in the cream.
9. Everything is finely pureed and prepared with nutmeg, salt and pepper and embellished with oil and herbs.

470 kcal/6g E/42g F/13g K

Spicy Parma ham with figs and mozzarella

This blend makes a heavenly dish.

10 mins

Ingredients:

- 400 g of Parma ham
- 240 g mozzarella
- 200 g arugula

- 4 figs
- 8 tbsp olive oil
- 4 tbsp balsamic vinegar
- 2 teaspoons of basil, chopped
- salt and pepper

Preparation:

1. First you wash the arugula, eliminate the stems and put it on the plates.
2. Then you wash the figs and cut them into bits of equivalent size.
3. The mozzarella is likewise cut into bits of the equivalent size.
4. Now you shape the ham into rolls and add it to the rocket.
5. The mozzarella, figs and basil are additionally put on the plates.
6. Finally, add somewhat salt and pepper to the plate of mixed greens and shower with a little oil and the balsamic vinegar.

655 kcal/40g E/47g F/16g K

Cauliflower rice with omelette

This omelet, in mix with the cauliflower rice, is especially filling.

20 minutes

Ingredients:

- 800 g of cauliflower
- 4 tbsp butter
- juice of one lemon
- 8 eggs
- 2 tablespoons of cream
- 2 teaspoons of butter
- 1 teaspoon of mint, chopped
- salt and pepper

Preparation:

1. First, you wash the cauliflower and finely rub it with the

grater so it is rice-like.

2. The "rice" is then positioned in a cotton fabric to crush out the liquid.

3. Then you liquefy the spread in a warm pot and blend it in with the cauliflower rice and lemon juice in a bowl and season with salt and mint.

4. Now you whisk the eggs with the cream in a bowl and season everything with salt and pepper, put it in a hot container with spread until it sets and afterward turn it

5. Finally, cut the completed omelet into strips and serve it with the cauliflower rice.

380 kcal/18g E/30g F/7g K

Fruity cream with fresh peaches

This cream is incredible as a nibble for the office.

5 minutes

Ingredients:

- 400 g quark, lean level
- 600 g normal yogurt
- 2 limes, fresh
- 240 g of new peaches
- some Xucker

preparation

1. First you focus on the strip of the limes and press out the pulp.

2. Then you center the peaches and cut them into bits of the equivalent size.

3. Then put the quark and yogurt in a bowl and combine them as one well.

4. The lime zing and the lime juice are additionally mixed in.

5. Depending on your taste, you can improve the cream with Xucker.

6. Finally, empty the cream into little dishes and enhancement all segments with the peach pieces.

125 kcal/20g E/1g F/8g K

Raw salad with fruity orange dressing

This crude vegetable serving of mixed greens carries newness to the table.

20 minutes

Ingredients:

- 800 g sheep's lettuce
- 400 g red cabbage
- 4 carrots
- 3 tbsp hacked coriander
- 4 tablespoons of olive oil
- 2 oranges
- 1 lemon
- some Xucker
- ½ teaspoon salt

Preparation:

1. Wash the lettuce and carrots and cut both into reduced down pieces.
2. Then eliminate the dry leaves from the red cabbage and cut the rest into fine strips.
3. Now you put the orange and lemon juice in a bowl and blend it in with the oil, the xucker and the salt.
4. Finally, set up everything in a bowl and combine it as one well

310 kcal/6g E/19g F/28g K

Coleslaw with lime and mint

A coleslaw can be updated with this formula, on the grounds that the mint and lime carry surprising flavors to the palate.

10 mins

Ingredients:

- 800 g Chinese cabbage
- 550 g carrots

- juice of 2 limes
- 8 stalks of mint
- some Xucker

Preparation:

1. First you eliminate the external leaves of the Chinese cabbage and afterward cut it into fine strips.
2. Then you clean the carrots and cut them into fine sticks.
3. Then you wash the mint, pluck the leaves and finely slash them.
4. Now put the cabbage, carrots and mint in a bowl and combine everything as one well.
5. Finally, taste everything with the lime juice and the xucker.

85 kcal/3g E/1g F/15g K

Roasted broccoli flavored with garlic

In this formula, the broiled garlic gives the broccoli an additional a scrumptious flavor.

10 mins

Ingredients:

- 500 g broccoli
- 4 tablespoons of olive oil
- 4 cloves of garlic
- salt

Preparation:

1. First, you wash the broccoli and eliminate the styles from the florets.
2. Then you strip the garlic and cut it into slices.
3. Now you heat the oil in a skillet and fry the broccoli in it, along with the garlic, equally on all sides.
4. At last, organize the broccoli on plates and season it with somewhat salt and, in the event that you like, some herbs.

259 kcal/10g E/19g F/9g K

Frittata with zucchini

You can set up this scrumptious frittata at home.

20 minutes

Ingredients:

- 200 g of carrots
- 400 g of zucchini
- 1 clove of garlic
- 3 shallots
- 4 eggs
- 3 tbsp weighty cream
- 2 tbsp parmesan, grated
- 1 tbsp rosemary, chopped
- 2 tbsp olive oil
- salt and pepper

Preparation:

1. First you wash the carrots and zucchini and mesh them finely.
2. Then you strip the garlic and crush it out.
3. Then combine everything as one with the rosemary in a bowl.
4. Now you whisk the eggs with the cream, the parmesan and somewhat salt and pepper and blend the combination in with the ground vegetables.
5. Then you heat some oil in a dish, structure level cakes from the vegetable mixture and fry them until firm on all sides.

360 kcal/54g E/10g F/12g K

Printed in the USA
CPSIA information can be obtained
at www.ICGtesting.com
CBHW030925031224
18319CB00059B/914